YOURSELF

AND

Your House Wonderful

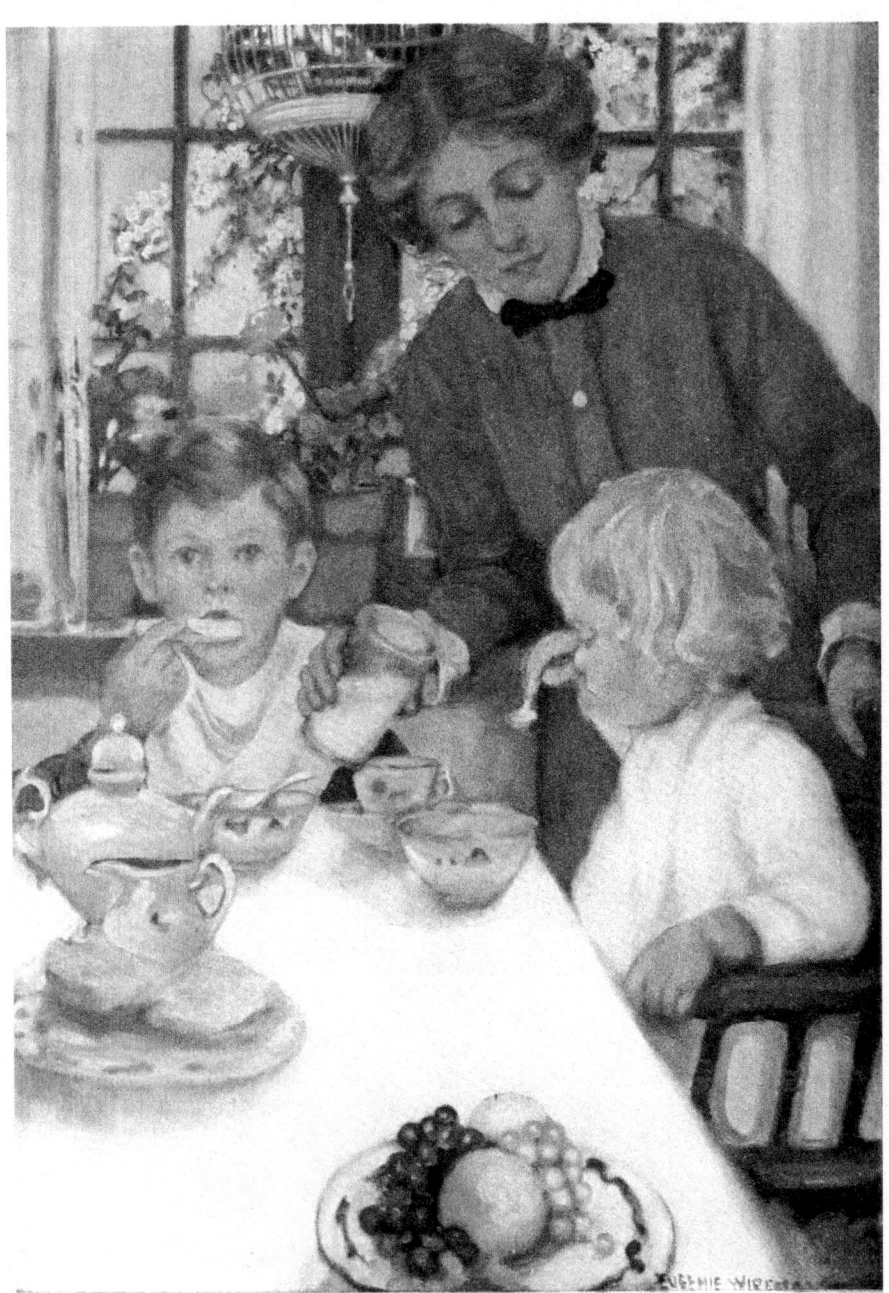

Work for the Stomach Dwarf

YOURSELF

AND

Your House Wonderful

BY

Hélène Adeline Guerber

2012
St. Augustine Academy Press
Lisle, Illinois

This book is an exact photographic reprint of the 1913 edition
by Uplift Publishing Company.
A new foreword, "A Note to Today's Parents," has been added by Lisa Bergman.
All other material contained herein is unchanged.

This book was originally published in 1902 by Dodd, Mead & Co.
This edition ©2011 by St. Augustine Academy Press.

ISBN: 978-1-936639-24-3

All illustrations in this book, including the cover,
are the original illustrations as found in the original 1913 edition.

DEDICATED

TO

ALL CHILDREN

WITH MANY HOPES THAT THIS BOOK WILL HELP TO

MAKE THEM STRONG AND HAPPY.

Books by the Same Author

Myths of Greece and Rome.
Myths of Northern Lands.
Legends of the Middle Ages.
Story of the Chosen People. (History of the Jews.)
Story of the Greeks.
Story of the Romans.
Story of the English.
Story of the Thirteen Colonies. (History of the U. S.)
Story of the Great Republic. (History of the U. S.)
Story of Old France. (History of France.)
Story of Modern France. (History of France.)
Contes et Légendes. I. (French Reader.)
Contes et Légendes. II. (French Reader.)
Easy French Prose Composition.
Joan of Arc; French Composition.

Märchen und Erzählungen. 1. (German Reader.)
Märchen und Erzählungen. II. (German Reader.)
Moni der Geisbub by Spyri; annotated.
La Main Malheureuse; annotated.
Marie Louise et le duc de Reichstadt.
Cupid and Psyche. (French Composition.)
Prisoners of the Temple. (French Composition.)

Stories of the Wagner Operas.
Stories of Famous Operas.
Stories of Popular Operas.
The Empresses of France.
Legends of the Virgin and Christ.
Legends of Switzerland.
How to Prepare for Europe.
Stories of Shakespeare's Comedies.
Stories of Shakespeare's Tragedies.
Stories of Shakespeare's History Plays.

Legends of the Rhine.
The World's Epics.

CONTENTS

		PAGE.
I.	Your Own Little House	1
II.	What Goes Into Your House	11
III.	Where Food Goes	30
IV.	Things You Should Know	40
V.	Your Twin Pumping Dwarfs	58
VI.	How to Air Your House	72
VII.	The Framework of Your House	97
VIII.	Your Pulleys and Ropes	110
IX.	The Outside of Your House	134
X.	Being Careful for the Sake of Others	151
XI.	Your Central Office and Its Stores	164
XII.	How to Train Body and Mind	178
XIII.	Good and Bad Drinking Habits	196
XIV.	About Smoking and Chewing	223
XV.	Plant, Fish, Bird and Animal Babies	237
XVI.	How You Came Here	260
XVII.	How You Can Grow Rightly	277
XVIII.	Your Companions	292

From the Editor:

A Note to Today's Parents
Concerning the Contents of this Book

In the world we live in today, with its rapid medical advances and changing viewpoints, one might wonder why anyone would be interested in a book about health written over a century ago. Not only has our understanding of how our bodies work become far more sophisticated, but many of the infectious diseases that plagued our turn-of-the-century ancestors are now virtually unheard-of. Viewed from this standpoint, the information in this book, along with the language and method in which it is presented, must seem hopelessly quaint and outdated.

No doubt this is true to some extent. Even young children nowadays are perhaps a bit sophisticated for Guerber's stomach and liver dwarves, and it is certainly arguable that some of the advice contained herein is no longer valid; however, the virtue of this work is not in what it does or does not contain, but rather in *how it treats the matter at hand*. And when we begin to uncover this aspect of *Yourself and Your House Wonderful*, we begin to see its quaintness in a completely different light.

To begin with, everything is viewed through the lens of a Christian respect for God's creation. Though the author personifies the various processes of the body as dwarves and servants and "blood boats", this whimsy actually serves to help us see our own body not as a well-oiled machine but as a group of individuals which must be carefully managed and treated with great respect. After all, not only are we made of a material far more temperamental than steel, our bodies are temples of our Lord, and ought to be treated as such.

Moreover, there is a beauty in the sheer common sense found in this book which is truly heartwarming. Some might laugh at the idea that children should not eat mustard, but the warnings about eating too much sugar have a well-founded basis in science. Likewise, few will begin airing their bedding daily because of this book, but we would do well to listen to its advice regarding fresh air and exercise.

But most of all, the topics of growing up, of making wise choices, of the proper relationship between boys and girls, and of reproduction are treated with a great deal of gentleness, perspicacity and sound advice. A very strong emphasis on purity of body, heart and mind are paramount. And it is this aspect which sets this book apart from any others. A parent can always supplement what their child has learned in this book with any number of excellent children's science books, but none of those science books will instill an awe and respect for the dignity of the human body in quite the same way. In addition, *there is nothing that a child might learn from this text that should be worrisome to a concerned parent.* The only regrettable thing I've found in its contents is that it reveals Santa Claus to be a myth. For Christian parents, this is actually not very troublesome, as we know that the secular fable of Santa Claus is merely a replacement for (and the namesake of) Saint Nicholas. Nevertheless, as many readers will have differences of opinion, I do strongly recommend that parents read this book before giving (or reading) it to their child. In this way, you may be certain that if your child finds any of its contents questionable, you will be ready to answer their questions as you deem fit.

Yours in Christ,
Lisa Bergman
St. Augustine Academy Press
November 15, 2012

INTRODUCTION

TO PARENTS AND TEACHERS:—

In conversing with earnest parents and enlightened teachers, who confide to me many of the problems which daily confront them, I have become more and more convinced of the pressing need of a work dealing frankly and explicitly with all matters pertaining to the physical, mental and moral well-being of our children. A book, treating not only of all the matters usually discussed, but also of excretion, sex, and reproduction, topics to which most books merely allude, which good people approach in fear and trembling, and about which none but the impure speak freely at all times and refuse to be silenced.

Our children have the right to know the exact truth about themselves. Were it possible and safe to leave them entirely ignorant and untrammeled concerning their origin, and all sexual matters, until adult years and mature understanding made full enlightenment expedient, I would gladly advocate complete silence. But such a mode of procedure has become impossible nowadays, unless we remove to desert islands. Whether parents and guardians are aware of the fact or not, the only alternative now left, if we do not wish to have our offspring at least mentally contaminated, is to impart ourselves, purely and reverently, all they need know. If we keep silence, through ignorance, false modesty, mistaken kindness, or innate inability to instil our knowledge of hygiene or morals, we are cheating the children confided to our care of their unalienable right "to life, liberty and the pursuit of happiness."

The difficulties of broaching certain subjects, are, I concede, considerable, but they are not insurmountable, as parents will see if they will carefully peruse this volume, which contains all that can help and will fully satisfy normal children. Pure-minded children desire to learn these matters in a pure and open way, and the mode of presentation here used, instead of harming even the prurient minded, will only serve to check their propensity to spread abroad such knowledge as they possess, by showing them how such matters are viewed by all decent people. Besides, it will supply the innocent with what they now lack, *i. e.*, a means of self-defense against insidious mental, if not moral and physical contamination.

There is, of course, much in this volume which all carefully brought up children already know, and nothing which they should not know, or which can shock any person who does not wantonly read into it more, or something else than it is intended to convey.

The last census stated there were in the United States more than twenty-four million children between the ages of five and seventeen, many of whom are less favored by fortune than yours. Educational statistics inform us that three quarters of

Introduction

the pupils who enter our public schools, leave at twelve or thirteen, and never receive further instruction of any kind. To fit such children—many of whom are worse than orphans as far as home training is concerned—to become useful citizens, and in due time self-respecting and capable fathers and mothers, is one of the main tasks set before us.

The schools have long realized that physiology and hygiene, once taught in the higher grades only, are indispensable at every stage. While from an adult's point of view there are now many admirable text-books on the subject, my attention was only comparatively recently called to the fact, that, from a child's standpoint, there is no work vivid, detailed or practical enough, to make so lively an impression that its teachings will ever after form part of the daily life of the recipient, and rise spectre-like whenever he or she is confronted by the temptation to violate any of the fundamental laws of health or morality.

As it is unsafe to postpone such instruction too long, this volume, designed for children under twelve, is couched in language of extreme simplicity, a very small vocabulary and short sentences being purposely used, so that they can read it understandingly themselves, and so that it will be perfectly intelligible even to parents of foreign extraction. A certain amount of space has been devoted to the care and training of babies, because many older children are constantly called upon to play the part of nurse-maid to their younger brothers and sisters.

Lacking the unsavory data which most adults have involuntarily collected in the course of the old-fashioned, long and round-about methods of acquiring divine truths, most children under twelve can and will see nothing more in this matter than what is told them here, provided they *first* hear the truth in all its beauty and simplicity.

A sufficiently detailed explanation is vouchsafed, to make them realize the sacredness and privacy of the whole subject, so no one need fear embarrassing questions or comments, and the knowledge cannot but act as a safeguard at all times and in all places. Besides, it will certainly put an end to further discussion of the subject with their companions among all those who are not already hopelessly perverted. The fact that such discussions are rife everywhere, and that the need of the instruction given in this book is widely felt, is not only proved by hosts of passages in many of the leading works on pedagogy, but was further emphasized in President Roosevelt's first message, wherein we find the statement: "The most vital problem with which this country, and for that matter, the whole civilized world has to deal . . . . is the betterment of social conditions, physical and moral, in large cities."

To effect permanent reform in these matters, it is not only necessary that each parent should take the matter to heart, and act as leaven in his or her own community, but it is also and especially incumbent upon us all to instil right views and principles in the children confided to our care, for they, a few years

Introduction

hence, will be at the head of all our municipal and governmental affairs.

This volume can be used without any restrictions whatever in the homes, and in schools where boys or girls are under teachers of their own sex. Still, most teachers are so thoroughly imbued with the desire to further the real welfare of their pupils, that none of the more enlightened women will object to read this book to young children of either sex, provided male principals have the sense and tact to know when to keep the class rooms uninvaded by visitors and to refrain from intruding, themselves.

My experience is that to most young children "all things are pure," and that one feels properly rebuked for all hesitation by the beautifully simple and matter-of-course way in which such information is received. Still, if the book is used in large or mixed classes, where teachers, often by intangible means, only, become aware of the presence of some vicious element, it may be well to set aside certain chapters for silent perusal, for home study, or for written recitation. A little tact and common sense is all that is required.

The perusal of this volume will certainly make a parent's or teacher's task much easier in matters which it is often difficult to check, or report, and public opinion among the children themselves will do more to enforce cleanliness and decent behavior, than any number of rules or the utmost vigilance on the part of parents and teachers.

Skilled teachers know that only through frequent repetition

lessons can be firmly implanted in youthful minds, and therefore resort to various devices to make reviews interesting. Parents reading this book aloud to their offspring will find the questions at the end of each chapter a help to fix the main points in childish memories, while teaching them to express themselves clearly. Extra zest can be added to repeated readings by announcing—as if it were some special privilege—that the first reading and questioning will be for the eldest only, but that the other children may listen if they choose. After a sufficient interval of time has elapsed to restore some of the glamour of novelty to the book, it can be re-read, ostensibly for the benefit of the second child, whose answers the eldest can correct or supplement when they are wrong or incomplete. With several children in the family this device answers every purpose, but with one olive-branch only, the reader can make a sort of game of it, arranging that reader and listener try at the end of each section to puzzle each other by asking alternate questions on the text.

This book has been submitted to the rigid criticism of several family physicians, as well as to parents and teachers of experience. The writer is deeply indebted to these critics and to many others consulted, for pertinent hints, and for help and encouragement. A few of the verbal illustrations used, have been drawn from the "Self and Sex" series and from the many volumes on physiology, hygiene, psychology and pedagogy studied with a view to present the subject in as broad, yet practical a light as possible.

As children are no more born with a sense for morality than with knowledge of geography and arithmetic, they must be taught what to do and how to do it. Earnest parents and teachers all over the world are realizing keenly that ignorance is not bliss, and that innocence and ignorance are not synonymous terms. This book is designed to serve as a manual for all those who are anxious to equip children to lead healthy, useful and noble lives.

YOURSELF

CHAPTER I

Your Own Little House

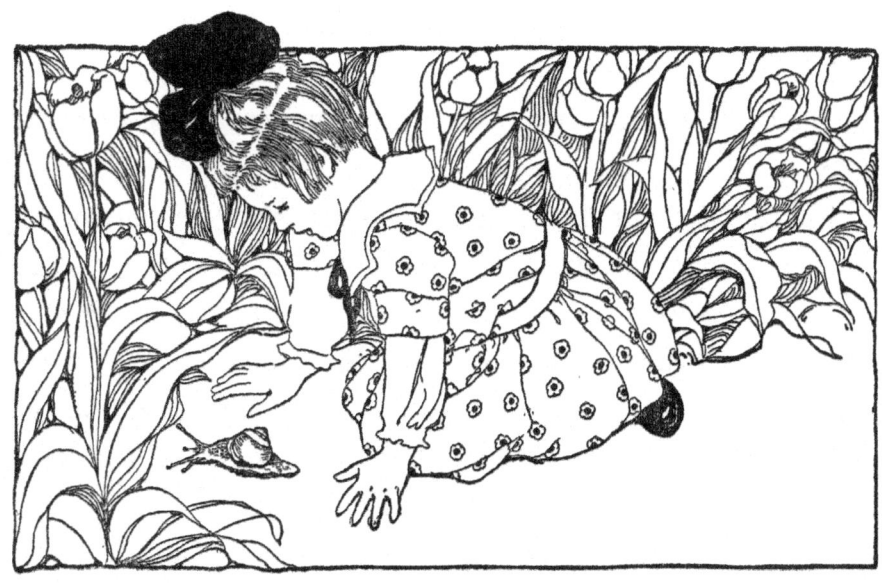

You Are Something Like a Snail

DID you ever think that you were something like a snail? Yes; you are, because you too live in a little house, which goes with you everywhere, from the moment you are born until you die.

This house is your body. It belongs to you, and you can

make it good, useful and pleasant to look at, or you can spoil it by lack of proper care, and thus make it ugly and unpleasant, besides making yourself very uncomfortable indeed.

As long as you were a little baby, your mother, or some older person took charge of this little house for you, but as soon as you began to walk and run about, you had to begin to look after it yourself. At first, nearly all you had to do was not to bump it against the tables and chairs, but every day you had a little more to do for it, until now you can take care of it for hours at a time when you are away from home or out at play.

Of course, your mother still watches over you part of the time, and tells you what to wear and what to eat. Mothers know that as long as you live you will have to stay in the same little house, whether it is nice and comfortable or not, for one cannot move out of one's body into a new one, as into a new house. So, mothers do their best to make their children's houses as good and comfortable as they can.

It is just because you cannot change bodies, that it is so important that your body, or house, should receive the very best care. Many children have wise mothers, who watch over them so they cannot do much harm to these little houses even if they try; but even the wisest mother cannot always be near you, and therefore it is right that you should learn to help her, instead of hindering her as I have seen so many children do.

When you are out at play, you have to take care of your

The Building Materials

little house yourself, and every child who is not an idiot, can and should learn to do it well. Sensible children can, of course, always be trusted to do what they know to be right, even if mother is not there to see that they do it. And, each year, as they grow older, they can learn to take better care of the house which God has given them.

It is because you have to look after your own house, or to live to be very sorry because you did not do so, that I am going to tell you many things about it. There may even be some things which mother does not yet know, for wise men are always finding out something new and wonderful about these houses we live in, and I have read many of their books so that I could tell you all you need know at present about them.

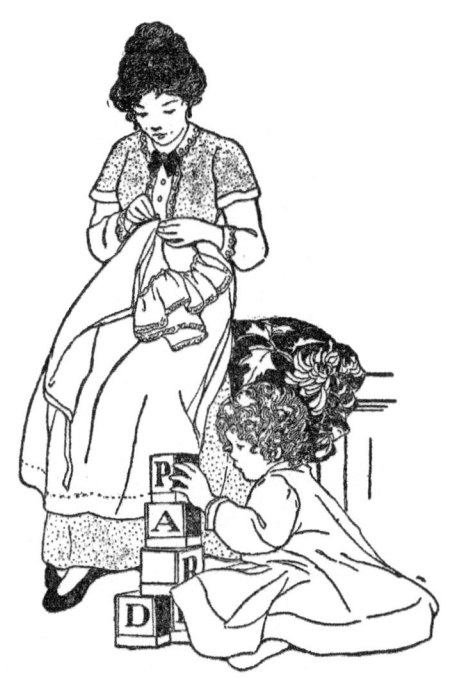

MOTHER WATCHES OVER YOU

THE BUILDING MATERIALS

The body is very different from the houses we build out of wood, stone and brick. Those stay where they are put, and are always about the same. But our bodies live, grow, and move about as we wish, and keep changing night and day as long as we are in them. You know that all houses look something alike; that is to say, they all have walls, roofs, windows, doors, etc. Our bodies, too, all look somewhat alike, for we all have

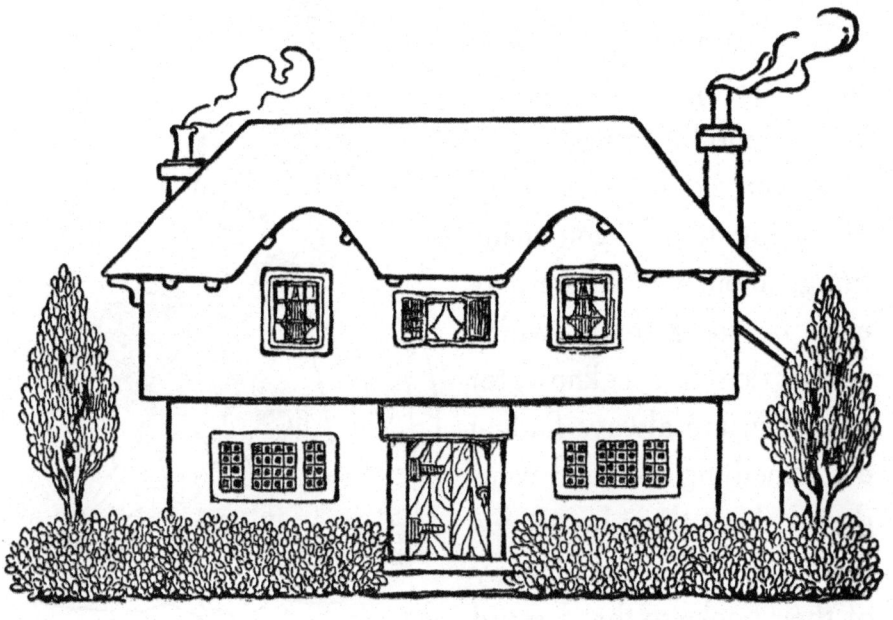

A Neat House

a head, a trunk, legs and arms, with eyes, ears, mouth, nose, and too many other things to mention.

All the houses you see are made of wood, stone, brick, mud, or iron, and when the builder does his work well, he makes good and pretty places to live in out of just these materials. If you want a house, it is, therefore, best to choose a man who knows how to build it properly, for he will make the best use of the materials you give him.

Wood, stone, brick, mud, and iron, change so very little, that a house once built, remains much the same for many years. But even a good strong house has to be kept clean, and nicely painted inside and out. Besides, new nails, boards, pipes, and plaster are needed from time to time, if the whole place is to be kept neat and in good repair.

Now, no sensible person ever dreams of using any but the right materials to build or repair a real house. If a window is broken, you get a new pane of glass; if a pipe is broken you mend it or get a new one, and if the house is dingy, you put a fresh coat of paint upon it.

If anyone were foolish enough to put a silk handkerchief instead of the pane of glass, to stuff cake or candy into a pipe hole to stop a leak, or to smear the house all over with molasses or butter instead of paint, you would laugh and think it a very silly way to act, would you not?

Our bodies are built too, not of brick, wood, stone, or iron, but of blood, which makes muscle, bone, nerves, etc. These, each house-owner has to make for his own use, out of food, water, and air. Since you have to make your own blood, bone, muscle and nerves, it is right for you to know how you can best do so, for there is good and bad blood, as well as good and bad bones, muscles and nerves; and whether all these are good or bad depends mostly on the blood-maker and on the kind of material he uses.

You admire good, strong and handsome men and women, and wish to grow up as tall, straight and good-looking as possible, do you not? Well, all this depends in a great measure upon yourselves, and if you will read carefully what this book says, and if you will do exactly what it tells you, it is very sure you will grow up far stronger and handsomer, than if you pay no attention whatever to the matters it teaches.

Unlike a house built by hands, the body, as I have already said, keeps changing all the time. That is because we are alive. Every breath we draw and every mouthful we eat or drink, works some change in our body.

If the air and water are pure and good, and if the food we eat contains the right materials to make good blood, to keep all the parts of our bodies in good repair, and to help them grow, all is well with us, and we feel happy and comfortable.

But if we breathe bad air, drink impure water, or eat the wrong kind of food, all cannot be well with us. We are then bound to feel more or less uncomfortable, and, if such a state of affairs goes on any length of time, we are sure to be ill.

The Master of the House

An empty house is very dull and uninteresting. It is the people who live in it whom we wish to hear about. If the house is well kept, we know that the people who dwell there are neat, and if it is pretty, we know they have good taste. We often judge of the people who live in the houses by the way those houses appear.

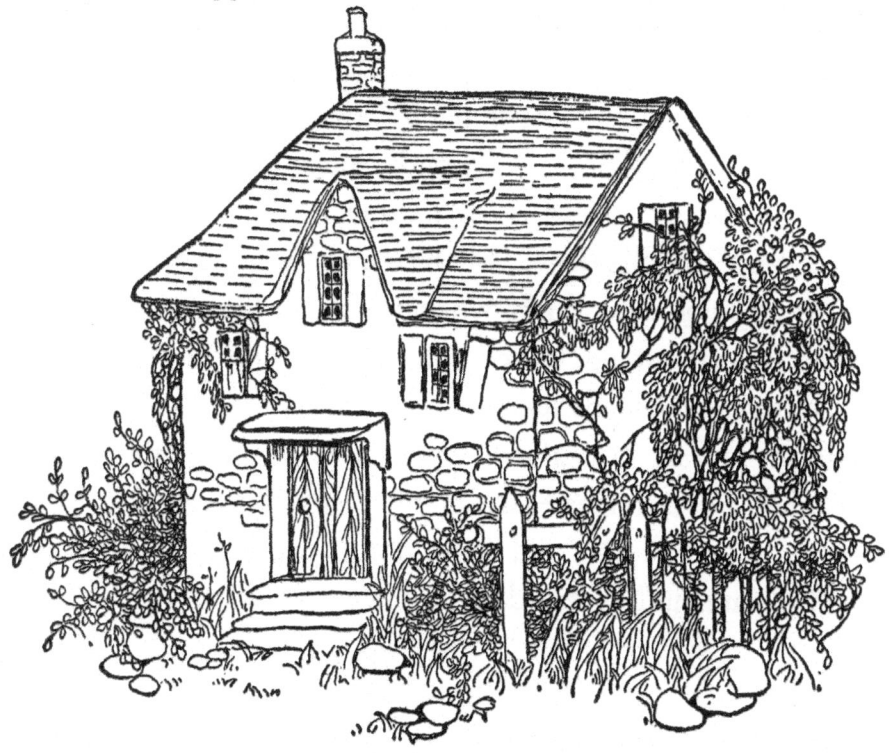

An Empty House

It is just the same with our bodies. The body is our house, and we would care very little about the bodies of others were it not that by looking at them we can often learn a great deal about the persons who live in them.

In houses, there are often many persons at once; some are

neat, others are not; some have taste, others have not; so, it is sometimes very hard to know just what kind of people are in a certain dwelling. But it is very different with our bodies. Each body has only one master, the real person, the part of us which *thinks,* and the body has to obey this master, who lives up in the top story, or the brain.

Each house-master looks out of two little windows—the eyes,—hears all that is going on by means of two little telephones—the ears,—and sends messages all over the house to direct what shall be done. He hears, and sees, and notices, all that is going on around him whenever he wishes to do so.

Many of the things done in and by the body, are done only when the master sends special orders; countless other things are done for him by his servants while he is sleeping or otherwise occupied, for each master has many, many little servants, all of whom know their duty and do it faithfully, as long as all is right and they are kindly treated.

The Front Door

The outside of the body is all covered with skin, in and under which run many little telegraph wires—the nerves. These tell the master of the house whether it is hot or cold, what we are touching or doing, and by means of them he sends word what he wants the hands or feet or any other part of the body to do. The skin is quite thick and hard on the outside of the body, especially in the places where it gets the most wear and tear; but in other spots it is quite thin and very tender and soft.

The skin not only covers all the outside of the body, but it lines all the inside as well. Still, the inner skin is not nearly so thick as the outer skin. In fact, it is so thin, that you can see right through it. You can notice this by looking into your mouth in a mirror. Your skin begins to grow thinner when it reaches the lips. It lines all the inside of the mouth and runs down into the house, lining the halls, rooms, stairways, and the many pipes which run through the inside of it in all directions.

The mouth is the front door of the house. When the master, from his post up near the windows (eyes), sees food coming, he telegraphs to the doorkeeper: "Open the door!" Then the mouth flies open and the food is laid down on the tongue, which is a kind of door-mat.

YOUR FRONT DOOR

The skin lining the mouth and tongue is so thin, that you can see the blood through it, and the little telegraph wires are so near the surface, that they can feel very quickly what kind of a thing it is which has been put into the mouth. They telegraph to the master for instance: "It is a piece of good wheat bread."

As soon as the master receives this message, he knows that bread ought to be chewed and mixed carefully with spittle, if it is to do the body all the good it should. So he right away telegraphs to the jaws: "Begin chewing," and to the tongue: "Keep turning it over and over." Then he also sends word to all the little spittle buckets, which are hidden under the skin of the mouth and tongue, saying: "Pour out spittle, keep the food moist."

All these orders are quickly obeyed, and soon the little nerves telegraph back to the master: "The longer that bit of bread is chewed, turned over and moistened, the sweeter it gets." Then the master answers: "That is right, that is just as it should be. Now, tongue, throw that food down-stairs, so that my servant the stomach can take charge of it."

QUESTIONS.—In what way are you like a snail? Who took care of your little house when you were very little, and how? Who takes care of you now when you are alone or with other boys and girls? What are houses made of and how can they be repaired and made larger? How can your own little house be repaired and made larger? Who is master of your own little house, and what kind of a master is he? Where does he live and what does he do? Can you point out the windows, telephones and front door of your own little house? What covers all your house inside and out, and what difference is there in this covering? Can you describe what happens when your hand raises something to eat to your mouth? Why should you chew before swallowing? When the food is chewed soft where does it go? Can you tell just what orders the master gives when he sees a mouthful coming in? What orders does he give to the tongue and spittle buckets, and why does he give them?

CHAPTER II

WHAT GOES INTO YOUR HOUSE

IF you look into your mouth, keeping your tongue down, you will see a hole in the back. This hole leads to a kind of stairway which runs *up* into your nose and ears, and *down* into your stomach and lungs. The part running down looks like two tubes. One of these tubes is used for the air we breathe, and the other for the food we eat. Instead of steps, these stairways or tubes have elastic rings which open and shut, as you can feel if you choose, next time you swallow.

You surely know that you can take in air, as well as food, through your mouth, if you care to do so. Well, the air-tube or staircase, is nearer the front of your body than the food-tube or staircase. In fact it opens just behind the hole you see in the back of your mouth.

When the tongue gathers up the food to throw it down the food-tube, which is just beyond the air-tube, the master quickly telegraphs to the little doorkeeper, who opens and shuts the air-tube, saying: "Food coming, shut that door!" Right away, a little trap-door closes the opening of the air-hole, and the tongue pushes the food back over it, until it rolls down the food-tube, where each step or ring opens to receive it and then closes behind it, so as to prevent its going in any but the right direction.

It is because there are such elastic rings in our food-tubes, that clowns at the circus can eat and drink even while standing on their heads! Although you might think that the food and water would then run down into their noses or ears, it all goes to the right place, thanks to those useful little rings.

At the bottom of the food, or back stairway, there is a little room called the stomach. This room, too, is all lined with skin. It is shaped something like a big pear, and is so elastic, that it can stretch so as to receive quite a large quantity of food at one time.

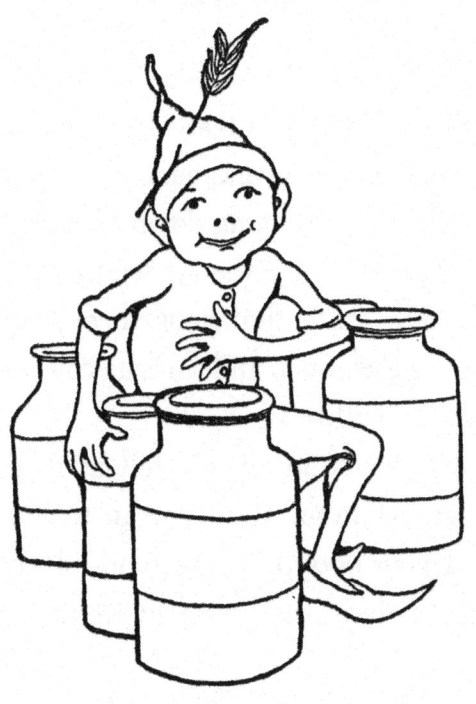

THE STOMACH DWARF

This little room is also something like a cradle or swing, for it rocks and shakes the food for one, two, or three hours, so as to mix it up nicely.

Now we are going to make believe (although the little room is really quite empty), that there is a little Dwarf who lives down there, because I want you to know just what goes on in it.

When the master telegraphs to the tongue: "Throw that food down-stairs!" he also sends a message to the stomach, saying: "Food coming, get ready to receive it." Then the Dwarf runs to the tube or stairway, and when the food drops down into the stomach, he looks it all over very carefully.

If it is good wholesome food, the Dwarf is greatly pleased. He rubs his hands with glee and says: "Bread! That's good. And nicely chewed, too. That's sensible. All mixed up with spittle. Ah! That is just the way it should be! That will make fine blood, bone, muscle and nerves!"

Meantime, the front door up-stairs has opened to receive a mouthful of meat, which the master saw coming too. Again he telegraphs to the teeth: "Tear up that meat!" To the tongue: "Turn it over and over," and to the spittle buckets: "Moisten it."

When the meat is just like pulp, the master bids the tongue throw it down the food-tube into the stomach. Again the air-tube closes, the food passes safely over the little trap-door, and rolls down-stairs, where the little Dwarf in the stomach receives it saying: "Ah! meat, and well chewed too. That is right! Meat should always be chewed up fine, or it gives me a world of trouble.

"I am glad to see that the teeth and tongue up-stairs are doing their duty. Master must have reminded them to chew that food carefully. Sometimes, he is so taken up attending to other duties, that he forgets all about it. Then the jaws stop moving, the teeth don't chew, the tongue won't turn the food over and over, and the lazy thing gets rid of it all by throwing it downstairs whole!

"That does make me very cross, I must say. I have no teeth down here to use so as to grind and tear meat to pieces. Then too, I like to have it well mixed with spittle, because I know it will be so much easier to handle, and will make so much better building material for this little house."

What the Dwarf Does with the Food

The little Dwarf cheerfully receives all the bread, butter, meat, vegetables, milk, water and dessert which is sent down the tube at meal times, provided it is, as we have said, nicely chewed, and well mixed with spittle. But he gets very cross when you pour a lot of ice water, for instance, down the food-tube. "Bother!" he says, "I do wish my master would not allow that! Here is a lot of cold water. Now I'll have to warm it all up before I can go on with my work. Why didn't he remind the mouth to hold it long enough to warm it a bit before sending it down to me?"

Still, the little Dwarf is, after all, such a faithful good-natured servant, that however cross he may get, he goes right to work to heat up the cold water. Then, from the sides of the stomach, where there are many little tubes, the Dwarf takes a

What the Dwarf Does with the Food 15

kind of juice, like, and yet unlike spittle. This is now mixed up with the food, which the stomach next churns up and down, and around and around, for one, two, or three hours, until it is all mixed up into a soft mass, and so changed that you could not tell any more what part was meat, or bread or vegetables.

Besides the little tubes which pour juice into the stomach, there are many others, which pump up the watery parts of the food after the stomach has churned it, and carry off this material to help make new blood.

When the stomach has churned the food for awhile, and as soon as any of it is ready to pass on, the Dwarf opens a little door at the other end of the stomach, and lets the soft food drop down into a big pipe, all ready to receive it. You will soon hear more about this pipe and about the food, but now we want to watch the little Dwarf. When he has got rid of all the food, he breathes a sigh of relief. He has been working very hard, and says: "There! that work is neatly done! Now I must see about making more juice, so that when the next food comes tumbling down-stairs I'll have plenty on hand wherewith to churn it up nicely."

The Dwarf then sets to work putting all the little juice buckets in order. Sometimes, while he is thus busy, and before he has had a chance to rest, the master telegraphs again that more food is coming to be taken care of. This makes the poor little Dwarf very cross indeed.

There are, you know, many children, who treat their Dwarf

16   *Yourself*

just so. They are very greedy, and never eat anything save what they like. These are often things which *taste* good, but which fill up the stomach, and do not supply much material out

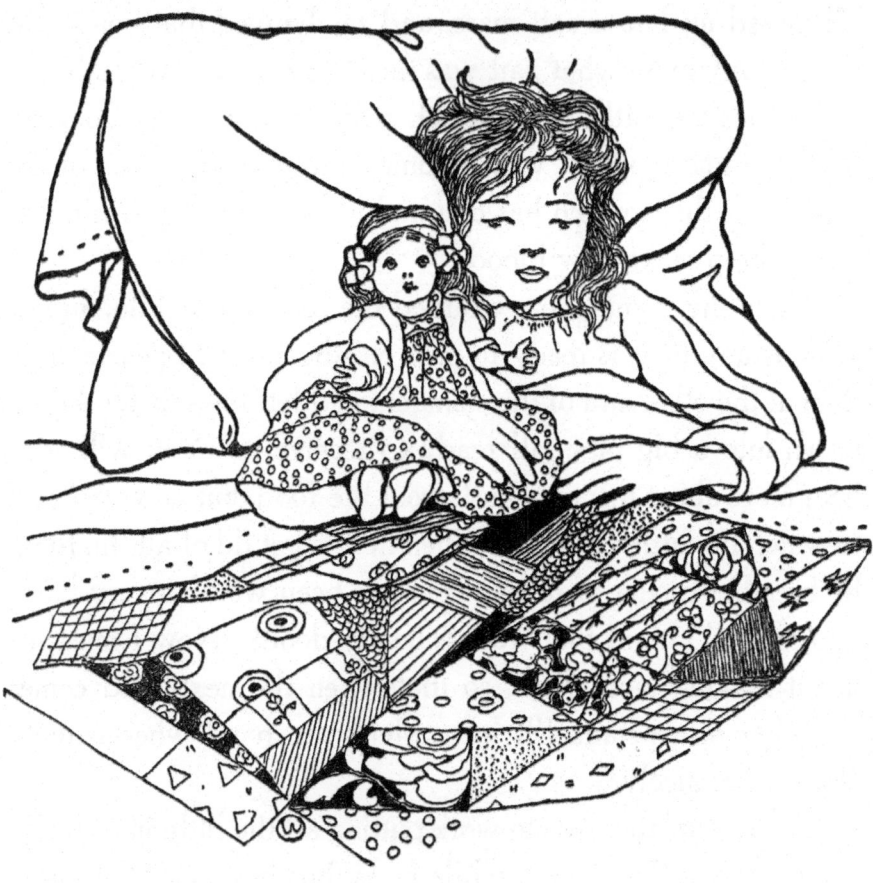

A Sick Child

of which blood can be made to keep the little house in good repair.

This naturally makes the little Dwarf very angry indeed,

for he knows he is working hard and all in vain. So he growls, and grumbles, and says: "My master ought to have more sense. Does he think I can make good building material out of nothing but candy, cake, jam, pickles, or such stuff as that? It is as silly as if he expected a builder to use loaves of bread instead of bricks, and taffy instead of mortar! Candy and cake are all right, if you only have a little of them, mixed up with the other things, such as milk, eggs, meat, vegetables, fruit and bread, but they are not much good if you get nothing else, I can assure you!"

When the Dwarf Gets Angry

When the little Dwarf is really angry, he goes about his work in a sulky, half-hearted way. He does not mix the food up well, and is in a great hurry to get rid of it. Sometimes, he is so very cross, growls so much, and makes such a fuss, that it actually gives the master up-stairs a bad headache.

At other times the Dwarf says in disgust: "Pah, food that does not make good blood always smells bad after it gets down here. Now I'll just let a whiff of the bad smell creep back up-stairs, so that master can know what a great mistake it is to send such stuff down here!"

Then the dwarf opens the upper door and the smell creeps up, up, up, fills all the staircase and hallway, and even rushes out of the mouth or front door. Then, other people can smell it too, for sometimes one hears them say: "Oh! Oh! So-and-so has such bad breath! Surely he has eaten something which does not agree with him."

As I have told you, the Stomach Dwarf is really a very good-natured, obliging little fellow. He will put up with much ill-treatment for a time, but when he gets very cross, and begins to rebel, he can make it very uncomfortable for the master of the house.

Once in a great while, too much candy or something else comes tumbling down-stairs which is either very bad for the stomach, or which is more than the poor stomach, however elastic, can contain. Then the Dwarf gets in a big rage. He stamps about, clenches his fists, and all at once he cries out: "I won't stand this any longer!"

THE STOMACH DWARF ANGRY

With that, he gives the stomach such a fierce turn and shake, that all the food which is in it is hurled up-stairs again with great force. The master, whose head generally aches at this time,—because of the noise the Dwarf has made, although no one else can hear it—now receives word that food is coming *up* the staircase!

As you know, this is not the usual direction in which food travels, and the master is horribly put out and disgusted at having things go wrong. Still, he cannot help it now, so he quickly telegraphs to the trap-door to close, and to the front door to open. Then the food, which the stomach would not keep, all passes out of the house again.

When this happens to a child, people say: "Oh, the poor child is sick at his stomach!" or, "Oh, poor little thing, how she vomits! What can be the matter with her? She must be ill."

The real trouble, generally, is that the child has ill-treated its poor stomach until at last it rebels, and takes its revenge by ill-treating the child for a little while, so as to teach the youngster to behave more sensibly another time.

When the stomach has thus been forced to punish its master for much ill use, it is just as well to give it a chance to rest. After a few hours of lying down, one can sip a little hot water into which was put a pinch of salt. This flows down the staircase and into the stomach, where the Dwarf is glad to use it to wash out his little room and make it all sweet and clean once more.

About a half an hour later, if the Dwarf is very quiet, and the master's head stops aching, a little warm milk and toast is very good.

Generally, the Dwarf receives this food very kindly, and if the master sends nothing but very plain food down to him for the next few days, he is likely to recover all his cheerful spirits and good temper, and to be once more the obliging, hard-working little servant whom I have already described.

The Dwarf Needs a Rest

Still, there is something besides wrong food or too much of it, which is very likely to put the Stomach Dwarf out of temper. That is eating too often, and you will see that it is quite natural this should make him cross, when I explain to you just how it affects him.

As I told you, the Stomach Dwarf receives all the food which comes down at meal times, and then sets to work to churn it up. This takes one, two, or three hours, sometimes even more. The length of time depends partly upon the *kind* of food which was sent down to him, partly upon the *quantity,* and partly whether it was *well chewed* and nicely mixed with spittle.

If during those one, two, three or more hours, a telegram suddenly comes from the master saying: *"More* food is coming down the stairway!" the Dwarf has to stop work so as to go and receive it. Then he has to mix this new food with juice, and shake and stir it up so as to get it ready to handle with the rest.

Meantime, the food which he has been obliged to stop working over, and which has grown very hot in the stomach, begins to spoil, and by the time the Dwarf can attend to it once more, it is partly rotten, and no longer good to make blood.

Then the Dwarf grumbles and says: "To think of all this nice food spoiling and going to waste, after everybody has had the trouble to get it ready and send it down here! Yes, it is a shame. It is good for nothing now. It won't make good blood, never mind how hard I try. If my master only had a little sense, he would have kept that front door tight shut. The very idea of letting in candy, cake, or any other stuff when I am still busy! He ought to

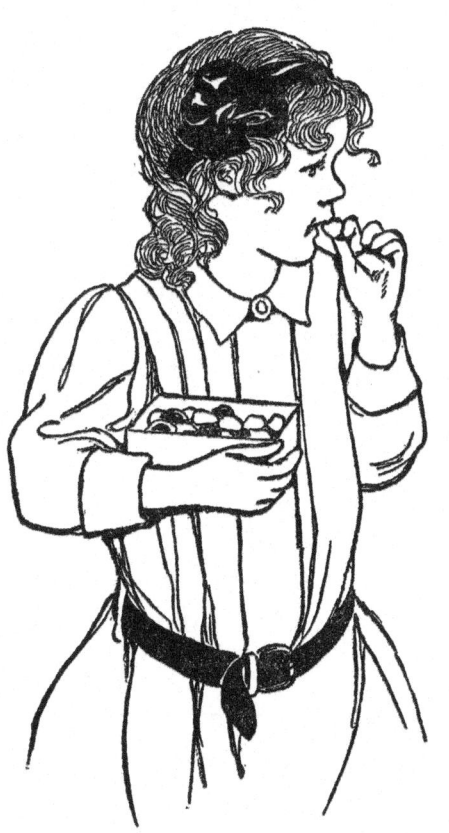

BE CAREFUL ABOUT CANDY

know better. If he does not look out I'll get angry and kick!"

Then, too, food sometimes comes tumbling down at the very minute when the poor little Dwarf has got rid of the last meal, is longing for a little rest, and a chance to make some more juice. This, too, makes him very angry, indeed.

Now, there are some children who *never* give their poor Stomach Dwarfs a chance to rest as long as they are awake. The little fellow is kept busy with a bit of this, and a taste of that, and has to work, work, all the time. Just stop and think how you would like to be treated in that way, and whether it is quite fair that you should treat your Stomach Dwarf so.

You surely see, now, why older people so often say to children: "You should not eat between meals!" Yes; the older people are quite right, it is *not* good for your health to eat at any but regular hours, and then you should take only just enough of the most wholesome kind of food.

If you are strong, if you sleep well, and if you have rosy cheeks it won't hurt you a bit to have a little plain cake, or candy, for dessert, but if you put sweets into your pocket, and all the time between one meal and the next, take a bite now and then, you keep bothering your poor little Stomach Dwarf, and by and by he will be sure to bother you.

Once in a while, a fruit stone, or a button, or a bit of bone, is swallowed by accident, and comes down into the stomach.

The little Dwarf turns this strange thing over and over, shakes it and moistens it, and only when he finds that he can do nothing with it, does he allow it to pass on into the big tube, so as to get rid of it as quickly as possible.

Sometimes the Stomach Dwarf, however badly treated, works on month after month, and year after year, as best he can; but he is nevertheless growing always weaker and weaker, and more tired, so that by the time his master is grown up, he will be quite worn out, and hardly able to work any more at all.

Then the master will always be more or less sick and uncomfortable. He will have to have a doctor, to take lots of nasty medicine, will be allowed to eat and drink only certain things, and be obliged to spend ever so much time and money taking care of a stomach, which, if well treated in childhood, would have grown stronger rather than weaker, and would have proved a faithful little servant as long as its master needed it.

How a Baby Should Be Fed

Until baby is a year old, at least, it should *never* have even the smallest taste of anything except the milk mother gives it, or the food carefully prepared for it in its bottle.

When most of baby's teeth have come through, it may have a crust of bread, or a cracker, to bite upon, besides having milk, baby food, and sometimes a soft boiled egg.

Little by little, as he grows older, baby learns to eat hominy, rice, oatmeal, mashed potatoes with gravy, and many other soft and simple things.

But it is only when a child has *all* his teeth, and when you can make him clearly understand that he must *chew* the food put into his mouth, that it is at all safe to give him even the tiniest piece of meat, or anything hard.

This is so well known by wise doctors, that there is a law in France, to forbid giving any solid food to children under two years of age. Any person caught doing so, is therefore arrested, put in prison, or fined, just as happens here when any one steals. In France they say such people are robbing the baby of his health,—his most precious possession,—and they are right.

There are some parents—who really should know much better—who give small children a wee taste of every different kind of food upon the table, just to see what they will do. These

A BABY ONE YEAR OLD

How a Baby Should Be Fed

people sometimes laugh until they cry over the funny faces the babies make. This is not only silly, but it is also very unkind to treat poor children so badly.

You all know how tender a baby's outer skin is. Well, the skin inside of a baby is very, very delicate too. It is so delicate, that the least little thing can make it very sore. Even a wee little taste, of one of the many things which grown people can eat without its doing them any harm at all, is therefore very bad for a baby.

Of course, after baby has once tasted sugar, candy, cake, and many other things which *please* him while in his mouth, he wants more. Poor baby does not know that there is as yet, none of the right kind of juice in his mouth or down in his stomach to mix up with this food, and turn it into blood, but the older people ought to know that.

That food goes down into his little stomach, where the Dwarf, who is all ready to take care of milk, or baby food only, does not know what to do with the strange stuff which has come down to him. He shakes it up, but that only makes the tender stomach skin very sore and uncomfortable. Then poor baby frets, and cries, and every one wonders: "Why is that child so dreadfully cross?"

After baby has been very unhappy,—and has made others very unhappy too,—some one may suggest that he has a pain, and give him a little medicine to stop it. But if baby had had nothing but his own food, and only at the right time, so that his stomach could have a little rest, he would probably not have needed this medicine at all, and would have been saved the discomfort he had to endure.

A baby who has never tasted cake, or candy, or anything but what he *should* eat, does not know that the other things are good, so of course, he does not want them, and he is much more likely to grow up strong and happy without them.

I have heard people say: "Oh, but baby sees me eat those things and he wants to eat them too." Well, baby sees you light a fire, ride a bicycle, sew on the machine, and do a host of other things which you would not dream of letting him do, never mind how much he wanted to do them or how hard he cried. And, after all, they are really no worse for baby than feeding him the wrong kind of food.

Even little babies can soon learn not to ask for or touch certain things, if the older people are only wise and patient in the way they teach them. If baby once learns that he *never* gets anything to eat, save what is put on his own plate, or into his own mug, he will not give nearly so much trouble as if he is allowed to taste what others eat. Some wise mammas know this very well, and are therefore very strict and careful, but many others do not know or understand this, and their poor baby suffers.

Sometimes, older brothers and sisters have to take care of baby while mother is out or busy. If you ever have to do so, you should be *very* careful not to give baby even a taste of any

What Hurts a Young Stomach

food *you* may be eating, because as you now know, his stomach is not yet ready for it, and you may make him very ill.

WHAT HURTS A YOUNG STOMACH

Until three or four years of age, a child's meat and other food should be minced very fine, or mashed, before he is allowed to

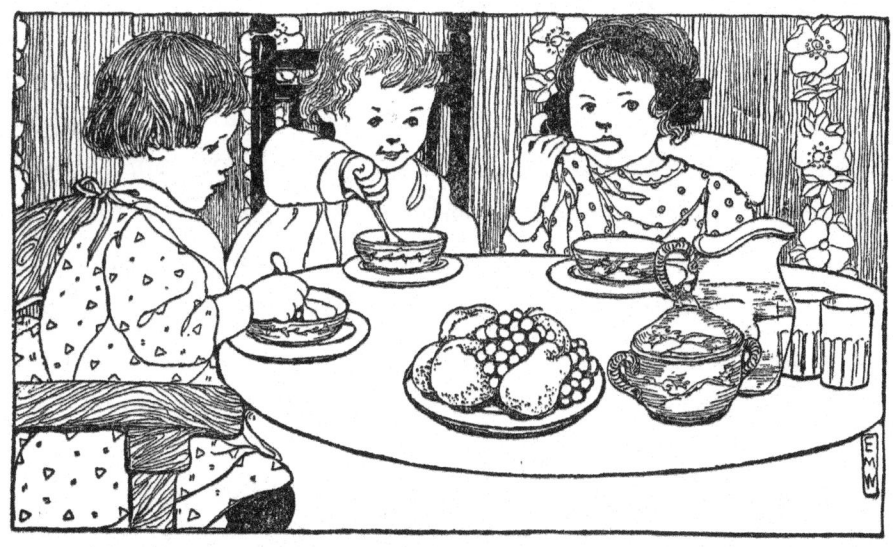

THE RIGHT KIND OF FOOD NEVER HURTS THE STOMACH

put it into his mouth. But, even then, he should be taught to chew it well. When he has learned to do so thoroughly, and when you are *quite sure* he can be trusted, you can give him meat which has been cut into small pieces, and it will do him no harm.

The lining of all children's stomachs is so very tender, that they should never eat highly seasoned things, and until they are grown up they should never touch tea, coffee, mustard, pepper, pickles or such things. Even then, they should use these things only very moderately, for they do not make blood and can do harm. You may be greatly surprised to hear this, and you may say: "Oh, nonsense, I have eaten pickles and mustard, and have drunk tea and coffee often! It has never done *me* any harm, and I like all those things!"

As I have told you, the skin lining your stomach is very thin and very sensitive; in fact, much thinner and far more sensitive than the skin covering even the inner part of your arm. Now take for instance, a small spoonful of mustard, just as much as you would put on your plate. Lay it on your arm, just above your wrist, and tie a cloth over it to keep it in place. Leave that mustard there, two or three hours—that is the length of time the mustard would remain in your stomach, you know,—and then *see* what happens.

Remember, just the same thing, only far worse, happens down in your stomach, for the skin *there* feels the effect of mustard much more quickly than the thick skin upon your arm. When you are quite grown up, and when the skin of your stomach has grown tough with age and use, a little mustard may not only do you no harm, but may even do you much good; but such things, while wholesome for grown up people, are decidedly bad for all children.

I have known some children, who, after trying the mustard experiment for themselves, and after receiving the explanation

What Hurts a Young Stomach.   29

which I have here given you, have been wise enough to give up eating all highly seasoned and spiced things, and drinking tea and coffee, although they were very fond of them all. In a few cases, the parents, not understanding the reason of this change in their children's diet, made great fun of them, said it was a cranky notion, and declared *they* had always eaten and drunk such things and so had their parents, some of whom had lived to be eighty!

All this is very true, but people who live to be eighty, in spite of eating the wrong kind of food, and drinking tea and coffee, would certainly have lived to be one hundred, had they done without such unwholesome things, especially while they were young.

None but very plain food should ever pass a child's lips, and certainly no child should ever drink anything but water, milk, or, once in a great while, a little cocoa, chocolate, lemonade, or some simple fruit syrup. *All* other drinks, even cider, root beer, and soda water, are *not* good for children, as will be explained to you further on.

QUESTIONS.—What kind of passages begin at the back of your mouth and where do they run? What are these passages for? Describe how the food is kept from going down the air tube. Why can the clown drink standing on his head? Why should you chew your food until it is soft? What does the Stomach Dwarf do and say when the food pleases him? What makes the Stomach Dwarf cross? When he is very angry how does he punish you? Can the poor little dwarf work all the time and be happy? If you eat often between meals what happens? Is it right to give a baby what you are eating? Why is it best for boys and girls to have simple things to eat? What is the food intended to make for the house? How does the Dwarf get rid of the food when he has churned it enough?

CHAPTER III

WHERE FOOD GOES

WHEN you go into a strange house, you generally see nothing but the reception room or parlor. But in your own dwelling you visit all the different parts of the house. You therefore know that you could do without a parlor, much better than without a kitchen. The kitchen is by far the most useful room in the house, and if it is kept neat and clean, one need not be ashamed to let any one peep into it.

Of course, when you have visitors, you receive them in the parlor, talk to them about pleasant subjects, and show them all the pretty things you have. Nobody runs for the garbage can, or the swill pail, to set it down before the visitors and ask them to sniff how bad it smells. Neither do you spread the contents of the trash-basket or of the ash-barrel out before your guests, or show them the soiled clothes of the family.

No, indeed, we keep only pleasant and clean things in the parlor, and talk only about those. But every neat housekeeper *has* a garbage can and an ash-barrel, and they are very useful articles indeed, much more so, in fact, than pianos or picture books. Our houses could not be kept sweet and clean if all the ashes, papers and dirt were left in them, and our kitchens would not be fit to stay in, if they were littered up with all the potato and apple parings, the cabbage leaves, corn husks, pea-pods, fruit skins, scraps of meat, bone, etc.

All those things would not only take up much room, and be in our way, but many of them would soon smell so bad that you could not stand it, and would either have to get out of the house or become very sick and die.

All tidy housekeepers brush up the dust, pick up the papers, and clear out the ashes, every morning. These are carefully put into the ash barrel, which you know, is emptied every few days by men hired to collect such refuse in cities and towns. The bits of food which are left over, and which can no longer be used, all the fruit skins, vegetable parings, bones, etc., are carefully scraped off the plates, and out of the pots and pans, and put into the garbage can. Then, a careful housekeeper covers it up tightly, so that no bad smells can creep out to poison the air. The garbage can, too, is put where the street cleaners can see and empty it when they make their usual rounds.

If you live in the country, each house-owner has to look after the house refuse himself. Some of it is burned, some given to the pigs, some put on the manure heap to rot and make food for the ground, and such things as bones and ashes are often used to fill up holes or make roads.

Now, although housekeepers or farmers have to spend a certain amount of time every day attending to the refuse, they don't make any fuss about it, and are not one bit ashamed of doing this work. They know that everybody has to do just that kind of thing, although it is not amusing, and there are far more interesting matters to talk about.

Still, once in a while, a farmer or a housekeeper has to teach some one else how to dispose of this refuse. Or, perhaps, some

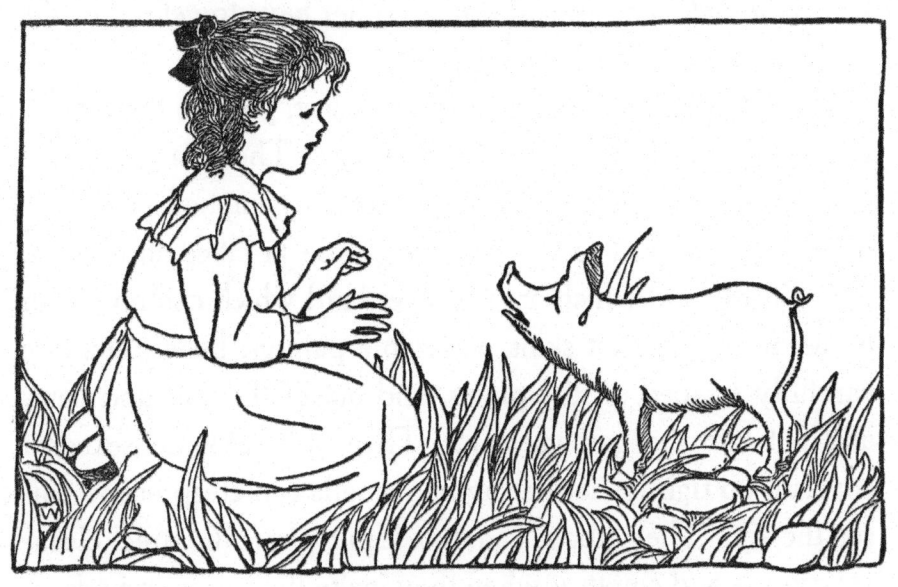

GARBAGE IS GOOD FOR PIGS

one discovers some new and better way to get rid of this rubbish. Then, he naturally tells his friends and neighbors all about it, so they can get through their work more quickly, and have more time to spare for pleasanter things.

A man, or woman, or child, who talks about refuse, with this object in view, is acting in a perfectly proper way, and if

How and When to Speak of Certain Things 33

he can thereby do good to his fellow-creatures, he is a public benefactor. But one who talks about it for mere fun, shows that he has a small mind, all taken up with unpleasant things, and that he is, therefore, unfit to associate with nice people.

HOW AND WHEN TO SPEAK OF CERTAIN THINGS

As our body is a house, into which food is brought every day, it stands to reason that while some of that food is needed to feed the master of the house and his many servants, there is a part of it which is waste or refuse. That part must be removed, like the papers, dust, ashes and garbage, which we talked about a little while ago.

Just as we are not in the habit of speaking before strangers of our ash barrels or garbage cans, we generally do not mention the body refuse in public. But just as an old housekeeper has to teach younger ones how to dispose of ashes and swill, so they can keep their houses sweet and clean, you must learn all about the body refuse, if you are to take proper care of your own little houses.

Of course, all children old enough to read this book, will readily understand that there are times and places for everything. If a subject, not generally talked about, is mentioned here, it is because it is right and proper that you should know all about it. *Stupid* children always giggle, snicker, whisper, nudge each other, and exchange knowing glances when such matters are spoken about in their presence.

But all the *bright* children are far too sensible to act in such a rude or silly way. They think: "Our mother or teacher knows what is in this book, and what we ought to know. We must read carefully and learn all we can, because our health and even our lives can be lost by lack of care in just such matters as these we are now learning about."

Of course, all the nice children know that while they must truthfully answer any questions parents, teachers, or doctors, ask in regard to this subject, they are *never* to talk about it to any one else. For although there is nothing *wrong* about the body's refuse, it is not one bit nicer to talk about it needlessly, than to bring the garbage pail into the parlor.

Now, I think even the smallest child who reads this book will understand how to behave, and I feel sure that none but those who have garbage pail minds will ever talk about it afterwards, save when they must, and then only in the briefest and nicest way.

If any one should begin to speak to you on this subject in any other way, you can quietly tell them that this book has told you all about it, and that you have far too much respect for yourself and for the house which God has given you, to talk about it unless it is really necessary to do so.

When the Stomach Dwarf opens the lower door of the stomach, the food which is ready, drops down into a big tube. As it has been mixed with the spittle and the stomach juice, it is already very soft. Still, it is now to be mixed again with two other kinds of juice, which flow down from factories just above this big tube.

The food which had already been changed by the mouth and stomach juices, is changed once more by these juices, and well shaken up again. When this is done it begins a long journey, for now it has to pass through many feet of tubing, all coiled up in your body, just below the line of your belt, or waist. This tubing varies greatly in size, and the different parts have very long names which only doctors are wise enough to know and remember.

Other people, when obliged to talk about these tubes, call them all bowels. Our bowels are very elastic, and they, too, open to let the soft food slide down, and close behind it so as to make sure that it will go only in the right direction.

The bowels are made of skin and lined with skin something like velvet. Now, you know that if you look at velvet very closely, you can see a lot of little hairs or threads standing up on end. If you were to look at the skin lining the bowels, with a strong magnifying glass or microscope, you would see the little hairs or threads which cover every bit of it.

Strange to say, every one of these little hairs is alive, and can move. Some of them pull the skin so that it will widen or tighten as the food passes, others bring a new kind of juice to mix with it, and the rest have tiny mouths which greedily drink up the liquid part of the food as it passes by. In fact, there are so many of these little hairs or mouths, that by the time the food has slowly traveled all along the bowels,—which are about five times as long as the owner of the house is tall—they have sucked up all that part of the food which is good for the body.

Nothing but the garbage, or refuse, is now left in the bowels, and that travels on to the place provided for it, which we will call the body garbage can. Even here, there is a servant, ready to attend to it, and from this place, too, little telegraph wires run up to the head so that this servant can send a message to the master of the house. If the master is a wise housekeeper, he attends to the matter right away, if it is possible to do so, for he knows it is not nice or healthful to keep refuse in the house a minute longer than needful, and he therefore bids the feet carry the body to the privy, water-closet, or toilet.

A good careful master, and neat housekeeper, sees that the garbage can is emptied every day at nearly the same hour, and generally as early in the morning as possible. He trains his little servant to be ready at the hour most convenient to him to see to this important part of his housekeeping.

But, if the master wants to have a well-trained servant, he must begin early, and not let him get into bad habits. Then, too, he must be sensible, and ready to heed any messages his servant sends. If the master does not pay any attention when the garbage can servant sends word that all is ready, the servant is very apt to grow careless and lazy, and before long the house is no longer well kept. Sometimes this servant grows so very sulky, that he does not send any more messages at all, although he knows very well that the garbage can is full, and should be emptied.

When he grows as lazy as this, it is very bad indeed for the master of the house. All the garbage which should be removed then stays in the house and poisons the air all through it. That, you know, is not right. The garbage or refuse which should have been emptied not only fills the inside of the house with bad smells, but it soon makes the master very uncomfortable indeed.

Then he feels sorry that he did not pay attention to the call of the garbage servant, who sometimes gets so cross that he won't empty the can even when his master tells him. When this happens, the master has to take medicine, or else he will be really very ill.

Why Garbage Should Be Removed

There are many, many children, who, not knowing how very, very important it is to empty their garbage every day, pay no heed at all when the garbage servant says he is ready. Sometimes they don't want to be interrupted in their play, and sometimes they are really ashamed not to have attended to that part of their work when they could have done so without calling any one else's attention. In those cases the master sends a telegraph message back to the garbage servant saying: "I really cannot attend to this matter now, just wait a little while."

Like the Stomach Dwarf, the Garbage Can Dwarf is really a very good servant, and only gets cross when badly treated. He therefore obeys this message without making much fuss, and if his master is sensible, and seizes the very first chance to attend to his work, he does not make any trouble.

But, every time one of his messages is really neglected, he loses some of his strength and interest, until he finally becomes lazy and unreliable. That is one reason why every house master should be so very careful about keeping him in good order. A properly trained garbage servant always calls to have his can emptied long before it is time to go to school, or to work, and then he does not send any more messages that day.

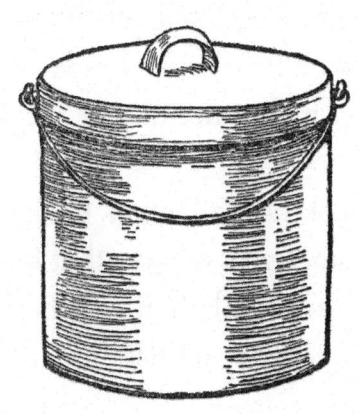

THE GARBAGE PAIL

But, if the house owner puts him off, or allows him to get into careless habits, the call may come at some other time. Besides, much more food may have gone into the house than is really needed. In that case, there is sure to be more refuse, for all food which cannot be sucked up on its way through the stomach and bowels, is waste, and has to be cast out of the body.

As every human being eats and has to dispose of refuse, every one knows that each house owner prefers to attend to this

Why Garbage Should Be Removed 39

matter when he can do so without attracting attention. But as every one knows, there are times and places when this is not possible, then the only right and proper thing to do, is to take it as a matter of course, and leave the room, or quietly beg to be excused.

Because it is natural for every living creature to get rid in this way of part of the body refuse, and because it is forced out by a squeezing motion of the bowels or a "movement of the bowels," it is often called by nice people "having a passage" or "attending to Nature's calls" when it becomes necessary to speak of this private matter to a doctor or to any one else.

QUESTIONS.—Why do you receive visitors in the parlor rather than in the kitchen? Do you show them what is in the garbage can? What is a good housekeeper, and what does she do? Does your little house have a place for waste? Is a house full of waste a pleasant place to live in? How do bright children act when private things must be talked about? Into what place does the Stomach Dwarf drop the churned food? Does the food go far, and how does it travel through such a long, narrow passage? What part is sucked up as it passes along? When the waste reaches the body garbage can, what should a neat housekeeper do, once at least every day? If the housemaster does not pay attention to the garbage servant's messages, what happens? If the garbage can servant sends a message when you are in class or company, what should you do? How should you call emptying the body garbage can to your parents or to the doctor? In what way can you teach your garbage can servant good habits?

CHAPTER IV

Things You Should Know

YOU have heard of the little tubes which suck up the liquid part of the food while it passes through the stomach and bowels. Of course, you wonder why these tubes take it up, and what they are going to do with it. These tiny tubes are so cleverly made, that they take up only the good part of the food, leaving all the rest. The food they take is all liquid and looks something like milk. They carry it off and pour it into many of the blood tubes, some of which go right to the liver.

You may never have heard that you have a liver, which looks very much like the liver bought at the butcher's. Your liver is a big, dark red lump on the right side of your body, very near your stomach and just above your waist line. It is a kind of strainer for all the food brought to it, and a manufactory for one of the juices poured into the bowels, to change, or digest, the food sent on by the stomach. Your liver, for instance, is said to take charge of all the sugar in the food you eat. Now, we are going to make believe that there is a Liver Dwarf, as well as a Stomach Dwarf, although you know there is really nothing of the kind, and it is the liver itself which does all the work.

The Liver Dwarf is very glad indeed when the pipes bring him sugar, for he knows it is good for the body. But, just because sugar is needed by all living bodies, there is a little of it in all of the fruit, vegetables, and grains we eat. In fact, there is sugar even in white as well as in sweet potatoes, and a great deal of it is found in carrots, peas, and beets, as well as in the fruits in which we can actually taste it.

The bread, fruit and vegetables we eat, supply nearly enough sugar for all the body's needs, so we really ought to add very little pure sugar to our meals. As I told you before, the Liver Dwarf likes to get *some* sugar, but whenever he gets too much of it, he has to work extra hard.

Like the other parts of the body, the liver is very good-natured at first. If the master sends down more sugar than the body needs just then, the Liver Dwarf thinks: "Ah, master knows I need sugar to make good blood. He has sent down more than I want to-day, but perhaps he knows he cannot get any at all to-morrow, and he does not want me to fall short."

Then the liver sets cheerfully to work to store away all the sugar he does not need, so as to have it handy for use by and by, when none is brought from the stomach and bowels by the little tubes. The Liver Dwarf says: "Yes, yes, I do have to work extra hard just now, but then my master will doubtless give me long rest pretty soon."

Sometimes it happens just so. But then again, it does not. There are, as you know, countless children, and many grown people, who eat a great deal of sugar in the shape of candy, cake, and sweetmeats, besides taking sugar in their coffee or tea, sugar on their oatmeal, hominy or rice, sugar, molasses or syrup (and that is all sugar after all) on their bread or pancakes, and even sugar on their lettuce and peas! All this sugar is more than the body needs, so the poor Liver Dwarf works over it, storing it away, and thinking the day is coming when all this supply will be sorely needed.

What the Dwarf Does with too Much Sugar

When, day after day, the master sends down more sugar than the liver can use, the poor Liver Dwarf gets very cross and tired and says: "This will never do. Here I am doing much more than my share of work, and all because master is greedy and selfish, and thinks that sugar tastes good. Well, so it does. I like sugar too. But, I like just enough of it. I don't want much more than I can use!"

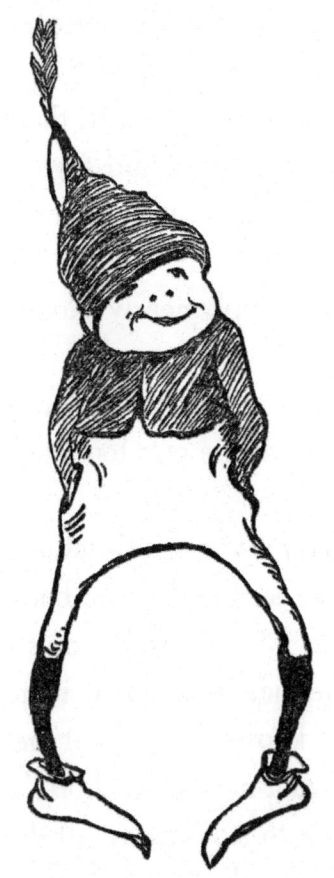

THE LIVER DWARF

What the Dwarf Does with too Much Sugar

After much ill-use, the Liver Dwarf gets so cross and tired, that he works slowly, and in a sleepy, instead of in a brisk, wide-awake way. Sometimes he warns his master that all is not well, by making such a fuss that the master's head aches, very much as it does when the Stomach Dwarf is angry. Sometimes he sends some vapors up through the tubes, leading to the stomach; they cover the tongue with an ugly white coat which looks so much like fur that people then say they have "furred tongues."

At other times, the Liver Dwarf sends some of his yellow juice all over the house, until it shows right through the skin and the white part of the eyes. Then every one says: "Why, how yellow you are, you must be bilious!" These people are quite right, for that yellow juice is called bile, and whenever it flows all over the house, instead of going only into the bowels,—where it is needed,—the body is bilious, and does not feel comfortable.

If the master is wise, he will stop and think whether he has been quite sensible and whether he has treated all his servants just as he should. If he is clever enough to understand what I have explained to you, he thinks: "Ah, now I know what is the matter. I have allowed too much sugar to come into my house. My poor little Liver Dwarf has evidently been overworked for many days. I really must give him a rest. What he needs is no sugar at all until he has used up all the store on hand.

"Then, if I move about a great deal, if I walk, and run, and

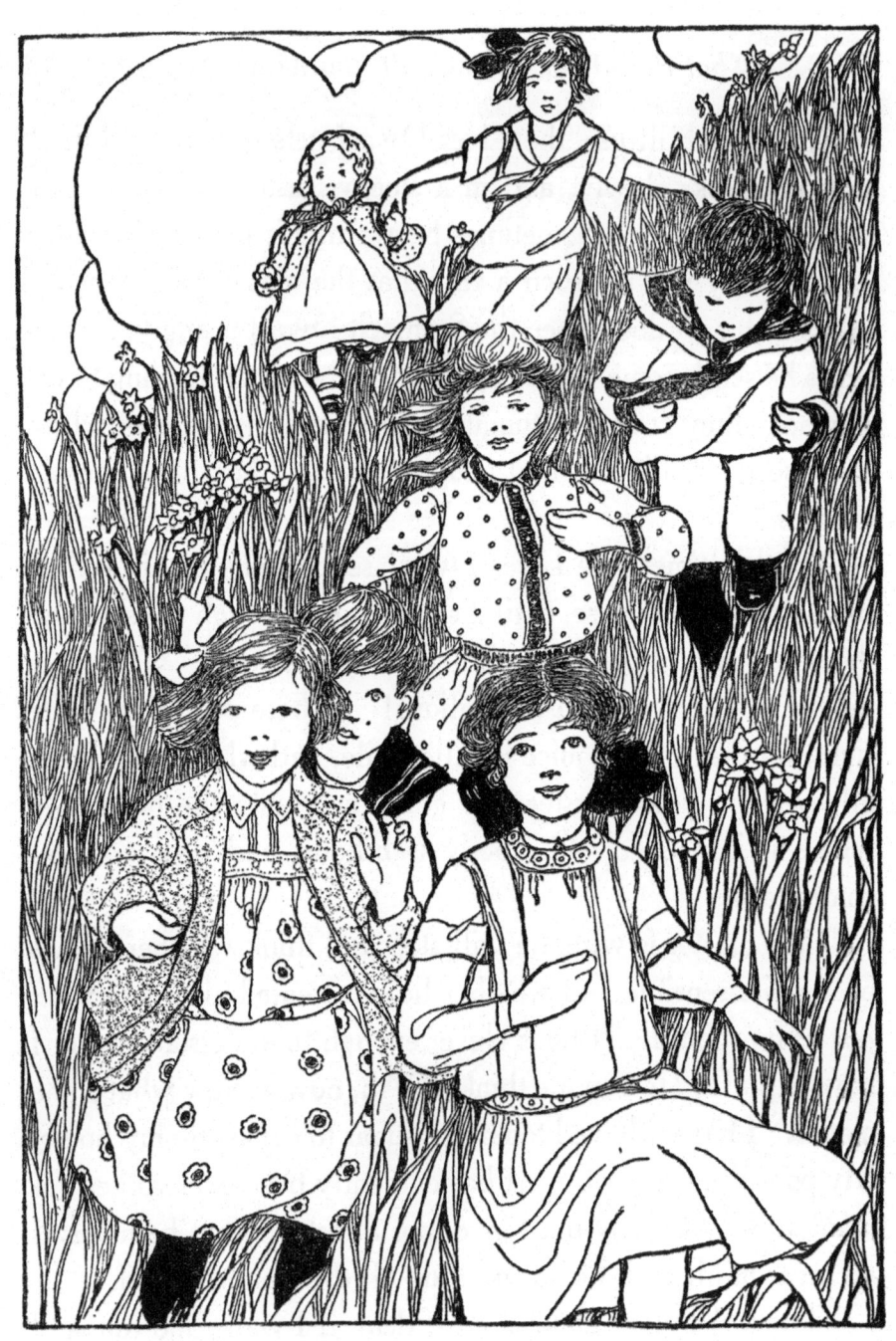

Running Is "Good for the Liver"

jump, or ride horseback, it will give my liver a good shaking up. That will please my little Liver Dwarf. He likes a good shaking, and will grow cheerful and lively again. By and by he will be quite ready to take up his work once more, and will stop making a fuss."

If the master keeps his word, the Liver Dwarf generally does get all right again, but if no sweets and plenty of exercise does not bring him around, the master should have sense enough not to take any of the pills or medicines which friends will recommend, as "good for the liver," but to go and see a good doctor. He will know what is best for this special liver, because all livers are not alike, any more than all people are alike.

The Waste Water

As you have already learned, all the solid part of the waste is cast out of the body by the garbage servant, just as in our houses we get rid of the solid waste by means of the ash barrel and garbage can. But there are other kinds of waste which are taken out of our houses by means of the sewer.

As we drink a great deal, and as all kinds of food contain more or less water, a great deal of liquid goes into our bodies every day. Some of this liquid is needed to make blood. But every day, part of the liquid in the body, having been already used, is no longer pure, and needs to be removed.

Nearly all the liquid we take into our mouths, is sucked up

by the little tubes in the stomach and bowels, from where, as you will learn later on, it is carried to different parts of the body to make blood. Sooner or later all this blood has to pass through the kidneys.

The kidneys are two reddish lumps, about as big as your fists, placed on either side of your backbone, just under your belt line. The blood, in passing through the kidneys, is carefully strained, for the kidneys are a kind of blood sieve. They are made so cleverly, that they can strain all the impure water out of the blood, and remove many tiny bits of yellow colored waste from it.

All the nice clean blood soon goes back to the heart, but the kidneys let the waste water flow down into a little sac, called the bladder. This sac is in the front part of the body, on a line with

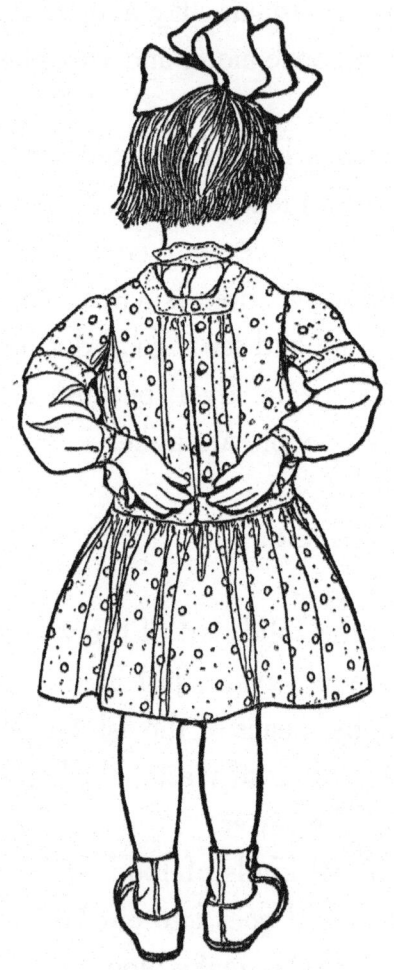

THE LOCATION OF YOUR KIDNEYS

the garbage can. When the sac is full, the Bladder Dwarf sends a telegram to warn the master that it should be emptied.

The master, who knows that this is true, generally pays attention to this message, and sends back the necessary orders to have the waste water emptied from the body.

It is because emptying the waste water is a very private matter,—just like emptying the garbage can,—that the body openings by means of which these two things are done, are always called the private parts. Nice people never talk about them, save when necessary, as I have already explained to you, and all except tiny children, filthy boys, and ignorant savages, always keep these parts carefully covered, except when they are alone in the water-closet or taking a bath.

Just as we must be very careful to keep our kitchen sinks very clean, and to cover our garbage cans, we must take special care of the private parts of our bodies. Every child old enough to read this book, should therefore get into the habit of washing these parts, every night and morning, with soap and water, for only in that way can one be sure to keep the house which God has given us clean as it should be kept.

What Happens to Careless Masters

When the master is too busy to attend to emptying the waste water as soon as the Dwarf calls that the bladder is full, he sends a telegram bidding him wait. The Dwarf obeys, but as the waste water goes on flowing down from the kidneys, his sac gets more and more full, and stretches and stretches, until it nearly bursts. Then the Bladder Dwarf often sends another message, so that the master will be sure to know how uncomfortable matters are getting down in that part of the house.

If this message also is not attended to, the waste water has to back up into the kidneys and stop their working. Then things are very bad indeed. The kidney servant is very angry because he cannot get rid of the waste water and strain the blood, and the Bladder Dwarf is angry because no one pays any heed to his messages.

Like all the other little servants in the body, both of these dwarfs have done all they could, and are hindered in their work merely by the master's orders. If the master cannot help hindering them, they are generally pretty patient, but when he does so only because he is selfish, or because it suits him best not to pay any attention to them, they get very angry. Then they take their revenge by growing careless and lazy, and doing their work badly, or by making such a fuss that the master often feels really ill.

So, you see, for his own comfort, the master should be very careful to see that the waste water is always emptied at the right time. If he is wise, he soon finds out that by emptying the sac, or "making water" as it is called, in the morning on rising, at noon, and in the evening before going to bed, the Bladder Dwarf is apt to be satisfied, and not likely to bother him at other times by interrupting him in his work or in his play to attend to his affairs.

Should a message come, however, in spite of all this, the master may be pretty sure that he is either drinking more than needful, or that there is something a little bit out of order in his body, and that he must be very kind and patient until the Kidney and Bladder Dwarfs get everything running nicely again. A good master can help them by being very careful about his food and drink, taking plenty of exercise, keeping his body just warm enough, and by not getting angry, for if one is cross, there is more waste water to get rid of than when one is pleasant and good tempered.

How to Care for the Little Ones

Most boys and girls have smaller brothers and sisters whom they often have to look after while mother is busy or away. In taking a little child to the water-closet, great care and patience should be used. Remember that if you keep a small child waiting, or if you do not give it time enough to empty the waste properly, you are doing that child great harm, for you are hindering the necessary body work from being done as it should.

Carelessness in this matter may ruin a little child's health for life, and may even cause its death. So you see how very, very careful you should be.

Besides using patience and being very clean in caring for little ones, you should teach them, as soon as possible, to attend to these private affairs themselves.

If you are always careful, if you teach them to do this as a duty, if you *never* allow them to play while attending to this matter, and if by every word and look,—as well as by the example you set them,—you show them how to be clean and modest at all times, the little ones, by the time they are five or six years old—or even sooner if they are very bright—will have learned this lesson thoroughly. Then, wherever they go, every one will feel sure that they belong to nice people, never mind how poor they may be, what kind of clothes they may wear, or how little else they may have had a chance to learn.

Most mothers, nurses, and elder sisters understand how important it is for little children to be taught these matters from the first. But a few very fond and foolish older people think that they can best show their great love for baby by admiring everything he does, by repeating his speeches, and by saying again and again: "Isn't our baby too dear, and cute, and innocent for anything!"

Yes, your baby is all that, and a great deal more besides. But if you wish to keep your babies dear, and cute, and innocent, you must begin very early to train them gently and firmly in the way they should go. If you do not, you may be shocked some day, by hearing some one call your "innocent darling" a "horrid, dirty little brat," and by discovering that this remark, however coarse, is only too true.

Babies cannot learn too early to be as clean and modest as babies can be, and whether they grow up to be nice children, and

What Older Children Should Know

pure-minded and decent men and women, depends greatly upon the training they receive during the first few years of their lives, and upon the example set them by the older children.

WHAT OLDER CHILDREN SHOULD KNOW

In our last pages we talked about the babies, and how to train them to be modest and clean. Now I wish to speak a word to the older children.

Never mind how poorly you may have been taught hitherto, you can all begin right now, to be clean and modest, and to train yourselves into right habits and nice ways of thinking.

No one, not even the most loving mother or the most clever teacher that ever lived, can train you

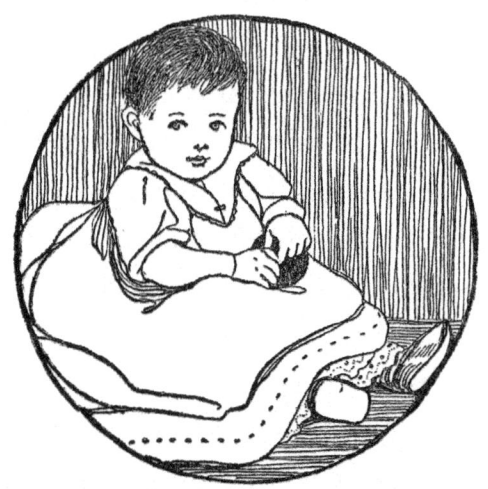

A SWEET, CLEAN BABY

half as well as you can train yourselves, if you only choose to do so. Whenever I see brave boys or girls take themselves in hand, with a mind made up to do what is right, I know those children are bound to make the finest kind of men and women. Because, such a resolve, kept ever in mind, is bound to have good results at last.

Such children deserve the respect of every one, and everybody should help them as much as possible. It is to the brave child, to the child who will do what is right and proper, even if some of its playmates and elders laugh, and call him "fussy" or "cranky," that I am talking now, for I know that cowards never amount to anything, until they change and become brave enough to face ridicule.

Careful mothers, who realize how easy it is to learn bad or careless ways, and how hard it is not to hear what other children may say which is not nice, always train their little ones to go to the water-closet alone, to close the door, and not to open it again until they are quite ready to be seen by anybody. These parents teach them that it is very bad manners to come out of that place until their clothes have been all buttoned up again, and everything is in good order about themselves and about the place they are leaving.

Some years ago,—perhaps when your mammas were little girls—it was considered all right for two or three little girls to go to the water-closet together, or for several little boys to escort one another. But now, all the careful mothers are teaching their children to go there alone. Before long, this will be so general a custom among all the nicely brought up children, that any boy or girl who seems at all careless in this matter, will be looked down upon as a very vulgar, ill-behaved child, be he rich or poor.

If you wish to avoid being considered badly brought up, and if you wish to do what is right and proper, you will from this

What Boys Should Know   53

time on, say very firmly and politely to any of your playmates who offer to go with you to the bathroom or privy: "Please excuse me, but I must be alone for a few minutes. I do not wish any company."

Then you can go in the bathroom or privy alone, and close the door behind you. Of course, if you have been in the habit of allowing other children to go with you until now, they may think this very strange. In that case you must simply tell them that you are never going to allow any one to go with you to that place again, because you now know that it is a strictly private matter.

Some of your playmates, and perhaps some of the older people who have not read this book through, and who do not understand why you do this, may make fun of you at first. But you may be sure that they cannot help but admire, in their hearts, the firmness and modesty of any child who will dare to do what is really right and proper, never mind what others may say. Later on, when they find out how *right* you were, and how *wrong* they were, they will be very much ashamed of themselves, and will wish with all their hearts they had never made fun of you, but had always been as brave and modest as you.

WHAT BOYS SHOULD KNOW

In the last pages we talked mostly about babies and girls, now we are going to speak mostly about boys. Every one knows that girls as a rule are cleaner and tidier than boys. That is because boys play rougher games and are careless how they look.

But, although a boy may not care how dirty he gets, or how badly he looks when out at play, he should remember that it matters greatly at all times what he is. He should therefore always bear in mind to be the right kind of a boy, so as to make sure he will grow up to be the right kind of a man.

When President McKinley died, every one in the United States whose opinion was worth having, thought that the grandest thing which was said of him was that he was such a clean-minded man that no one ever ventured to tell a bad story or make any improper remark in his presence.

This, I am happy to say, is true of many men in our country. But then, too, there are many really pure-minded men here, who are not as brave as McKinley, and who do not dare to show others by their looks, their manner, or when necessary, by a few brief words, that they will not allow others to use improper words or to mention improper or private things in their hearing.

McKinley did not wait until he was President of the United States to show his dislike for all such low, ill-bred things. He had begun long, long before that. A clean-minded man could only have been a clean-minded boy; one who loved and respected his mother, and who was not willing to do or hear anything which he would not like her to know.

Boys who wish to grow up to deserve such high praise as that, must begin right now. Although every boy cannot become

President, all boys can be good, true, clean-minded men, if they choose to do so.

A boy who wishes to grow up to deserve the respect of everybody must begin by respecting himself, and he can do so only when his conscience tells him that he is doing what is right and that he is worthy of respect.

Even a boy of five ought to know that he must attend to the calls of the garbage can and the waste water dwarfs only in private. Whenever it is possible, he should, even at the cost of some time and trouble, go to the place provided for that purpose. Many boys are far from careful or modest about this matter, but if they knew what older people, and especially what girls and women think of their carelessness, they would blush redder than any flower that ever grew, and hide their heads in bitter shame.

When they are still very little, people blame their *mothers* severely, but you can easily imagine how shocked and mortified some of those poor mothers would be, if they knew that their dear boys were behaving more like dogs than like human beings!

When such careless boys grow up, they are likely to forget themselves, merely because they have gotten into bad habits. That is the reason why there are so many men whom gentlemanly men call brutes, although the brutes are really not half as bad, for they know no better.

Another thing which boys should be more careful about, is getting undressed on the bank of a river or brook, and going in swimming without bathing tights. In cities, boys who are of so low a class, and so lost to all sense of decency and shame as to do that, are arrested.

In country towns, where policemen are few, those who offend thus against the laws of decency, are seldom punished. That is to say, they are not arrested, but I know of more than one boy who is no longer invited to certain nice houses, simply because some older member of the family learned that he was not careful enough in these matters to be trustworthy.

It is not always easy for a boy to find a house near the river or pond, where he *can* undress. But every boy can look carefully around, to make sure he is not in sight of any house or any party of pleasure seekers.

Besides, he can surely find a clump of bushes, a pile of lumber, a heap of rocks, or a tree trunk, behind which he can stand

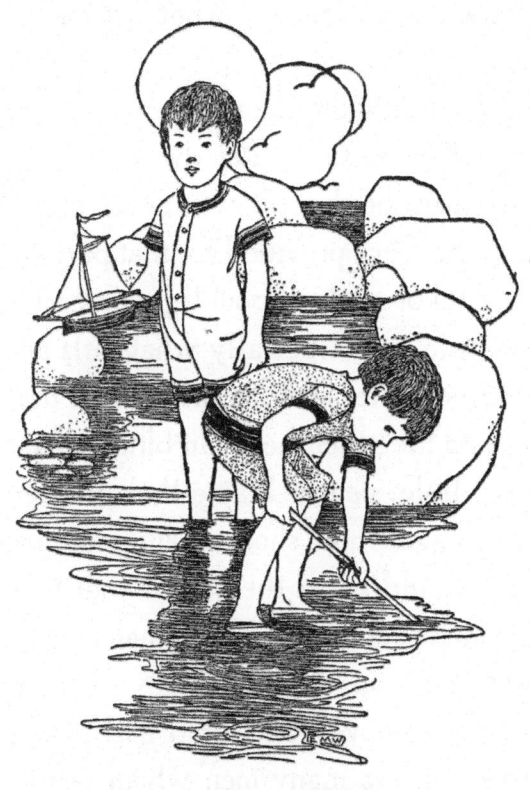

GOOD COSTUMES FOR BATHING

What Boys Should Know

while undressing and dressing. It is always easy for a boy to carry his bathing tights in his pocket, and a boy who goes in bathing without them, in any place where he is at all likely to be seen by any one, shows that he has none of the fine feelings which go to make a gentleman.

There are some men who merely laugh at such matters and say: "Oh! Boys will be boys." But gentlemanly men declare that "Boys can be boys, but they do not need to be pigs!" Yes; you can be boys, and nice boys too, and can have plenty of the kind of fun that will always linger in your minds without bringing a blush to your cheeks. But the only way to do so, is to remember *never* to do anything which you would not be willing to tell your mother or to let her see.

QUESTIONS.—How does your food get into your blood? Where and what is your liver? What does the Liver Dwarf like? When too much sugar is sent to the Liver Dwarf, what does he do? In what part of your body is the blood strained? Where does the good part go? Where does the bad part go? How does the Bladder Dwarf get rid of it? How does the Bladder Dwarf punish a careless housekeeper? How can you train your Bladder Dwarf into good habits? When you take little brothers and sisters to the water-closet, should you be patient, and what should you teach them? Is it nice for big children to go to the water-closet with others? When boys attend to Nature's calls in public, or undress for a swim in everybody's sight, what do well-bred people think?

CHAPTER V

YOUR TWIN PUMPING DWARFS

YOU have already heard of several of the clever little servants who live in your house and work for you night and day as long as you live. They do not ask for any wages or holidays, and keep cheerful and active as long as you treat them kindly, and do not hinder them too much in their work.

Now I am going to tell you about the Twin Dwarfs, who live in the pumping station. They, too, are very busy little servants, and if you put your ear down on any one's chest, just a little below the left breast, you can easily hear these two little dwarfs working busily night and day.

The pumping station is also called the heart. Although it is only as big as your fist, it is divided into four small rooms, in which a great deal of work is done, as you are going to see. There is a thin but strong wall running right through the middle of the heart, or pumping station, and as there is no opening of any kind in this wall, the twins, who live on either side of it, never catch a glimpse of each other. Still, they can hear each other, exchange telegrams, and their duties are so very much alike that they are real twins in every way.

Your Twin Pumping Dwarfs 59

On the left side of the heart, at the top there is a room, (auricle) into which a pipe pours bright, red blood. When this room is full of blood, the Pumping Dwarf, who lives on that side of the heart, opens a little trap-door in the floor and lets the blood flow down into a room just below it, (ventricle) whose walls are very elastic indeed.

When all the blood has flowed down, the Dwarf closes the door again, and begins to tug at some ropes which draw that elastic walled room together, very much in the same way as you squeeze a rubber bulb in your hand.

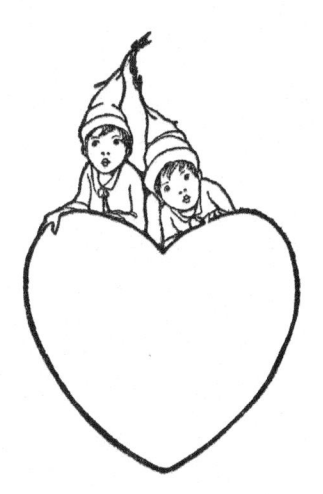

THE PUMPING TWINS

Of course, the blood which the room contains has to go somewhere, and as the doors above are shut tight, and it cannot go back into the upper room, it rushes quickly down into a big pipe in one corner of the lower room, making a roaring noise which you can hear if you listen very closely with your ear against some one's chest.

The blood thus forced out of the lower room by Pumping Dwarf number one, flows swiftly along the big tube which soon divides into two smaller branches. These, in turn, break up into two more, which both split up before long, and so it goes on, each tube being just a little smaller than the one before, until at last the tubes get to be finer than the finest hair.

When the Pumping Dwarf has emptied his lower chamber, he takes a wee rest while the upper chamber fills up once more. Then he starts up, opens the door, closes it again, tugs at his ropes, and sends a new roomful of blood down into the big tube.

Night and day the Pumping Dwarf works, resting only between each squeeze, and he is so steady and reliable that you can hear him working away almost as regularly as a clock ticks. He is so faithful, that the master does not need to remind him of his duty, or to send him any orders. In fact, the master can go to sleep, feeling quite sure the Pumping Dwarf will go on working just as steadily as if he were watched every minute.

The Pumping Dwarf works on so steadily, not only because he is a good servant, but because he knows that new blood is needed in all the different parts of the body every second. He is aware of the fact that you need more blood when you are running, than when you are sitting still, and more when you are awake than when you are asleep; so he pumps more or less fast to keep up the supply.

THE BLOOD-BOATS

You may wonder why it is so very important that fresh blood should go to all parts of the body so often, and I am going to try and explain it so that you will be sure to understand. You have all seen blood, and so you all know that it *looks* very much like bright red water. Still, none of you have sharp enough eyes

The Blood-Boats

to see what wise doctors have found out by means of their microscopes. That is that blood is really made of several things.

Here is a little glass bottle. It is quite empty so you can see right through it. Now I am going to fill it with pure water. You can still see through the bottle, can you not? And, if I hold it far enough away, you cannot feel quite sure whether it it is full or empty, because clear water and clean glass look very much alike at a distance.

I am now going to drop all these tiny red glass beads into the bottle. See, it is quite full of them, although there is still a little water between and around the beads. If I hold the bottle far enough away from you, you won't notice the water at all, but the bottle will look just as if it were filled with some red liquid.

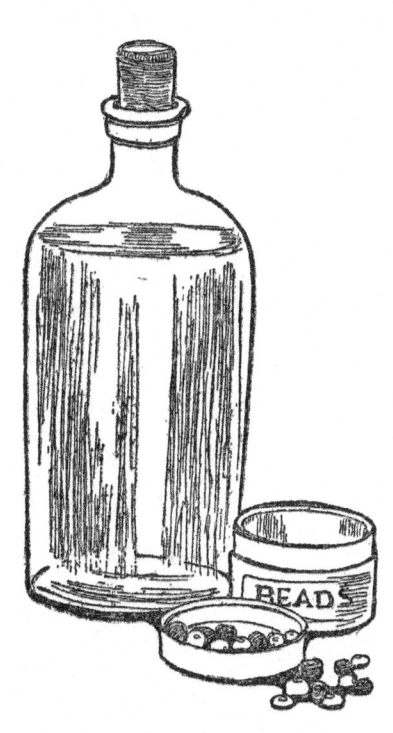

THE BOTTLE AND BEADS

Next, we will empty the bottle, and fill it again with water and red beads, but putting in one white glass bead to every three hundred red ones. If I hold the bottle far away, you won't notice either the water or the white beads, and it will still look just as if the bottle were full of red liquid. But, if I bring it near enough to your eyes, you will be able to see the water, and even to count the red and white beads.

It is just the same with our blood. All the blood in our bodies is made up of a yellowish kind of water, in which float many, many red and white things shaped something like beads. The red ones are so many, and lie so close together in the yellow water, that they make it look red, just as the water in the bottle looked red when many red beads were in it, and I held it at a distance.

The little red beads in the blood are so very tiny, that no human eye has ever been sharp enough to see them, but a microscope shows them very plainly. As you know, the red and white glass beads in the bottle are all hard and lifeless, but each of the little red or white beads in our blood is soft and alive. In fact, each one of them is something like a little boat, for it floats rapidly along in the watery part of the blood, carrying a load of food and air to all the different parts of the body.

Since the blood beads or boats are so very small that you cannot see them without the help of a microscope, you can readily understand what very small loads of food and air they carry. But, there are so very many of them, and they travel so *very* fast, that small as they are, they manage to carry plenty of food, air, and other building materials to all parts of the body, so that it can be kept in good repair and even be made to grow.

How the Blood-Boats Load and Unload

The little blood-boats are so clever at loading and unloading, that they can give up all their good food and air, and take up the waste material and bad air in exchange, without stopping long enough for us to notice it. Besides, they float along so swiftly, that wise doctors have found out it takes much less than five minutes for the blood-boats to sail through many, many feet of tubing, reach the furthest part of the body, unload, load up again, and get back to their starting-place.

You have heard how the big tube, starting from the heart, divides up again and again. The blood-ships, instead of sailing ever so many side by side in a broad river,

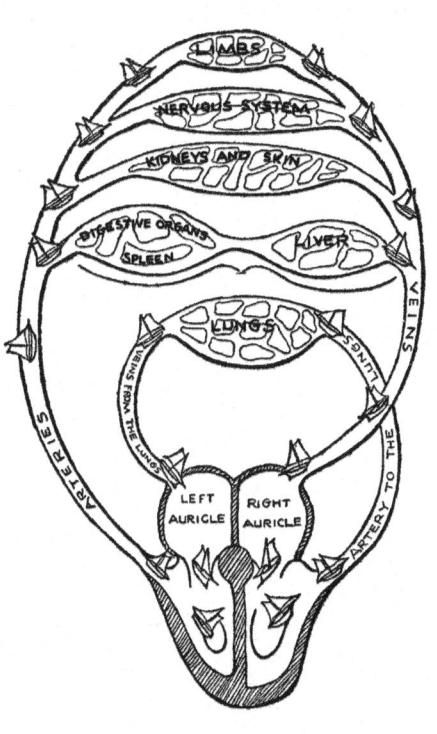

CIRCULATION AND BLOOD BOATS

finally have to pass single file down tiny canals. In fact some blood canals are so tiny, and they are so numerous, that you can hardly run the finest needle into any part of your body without piercing one of them, and thus causing blood to flow out.

After the pipes leading *from* the heart (the arteries) have divided up until they cannot divide any more, the blood-boats pass into a new set of pipes (the veins), which do just the contrary. They are tiny and numerous at first, but two keep joining into one, until they get bigger and bigger, as they draw near the heart once more. All the blood-boats which were sent out from the heart always come back to it after giving up their loads of air and food. They come back laden with bad air and refuse, and meet many other boats coming up from the liver and bowels laden with food to use.

As you know, a ship leaving port is generally freshly painted, neat and clean, and fully loaded. But a ship coming back to port, after a long journey, often looks dingy, battered and untidy. Before it can start out on a new journey, it needs to be repaired, cleaned and painted,—or overhauled as sailors generally call it.

It is just the same with the little ships in our blood. They are clean and look bright and red when they begin their journey; but by the time they have carried their cargo to the place where it belongs, and brought back a load of refuse, they are so battered and dirty and dingy, that the stream in which they float, instead of looking bright red, seems dark red or purplish in hue.

In fact, the change in the color of the little blood-ships is so great, that people generally say that the blood which Dwarf Number One sends out is red while the blood which comes back to Dwarf Number Two is blue.

PUMPING DWARF NUMBER TWO

When the blood-ships come back dingy, worn and laden with refuse, the stream in which they float pours right down into the top room on the right side of the heart wall. When this room is full of blood, the second Twin Dwarf opens his trap-door in the floor, and lets it flow down into the lower room. This is exactly like the room on the other side of the wall, and Dwarf Number Two also has ropes to pull so that he can squeeze the bluish blood into a big pipe too.

But, this time, it is dirty blood which flows out, and before it can do any more work it has to be cleaned. The place where this is done is the lungs, about which we will talk more further on. Just now, it is enough for you to know that in the lungs, each little ship will not only be cleaned and repaired, but relieved of its load of refuse, given nice fresh air and food to carry, and sent back to the Pumping Station, where Dwarf Number One will start it out again on a new journey.

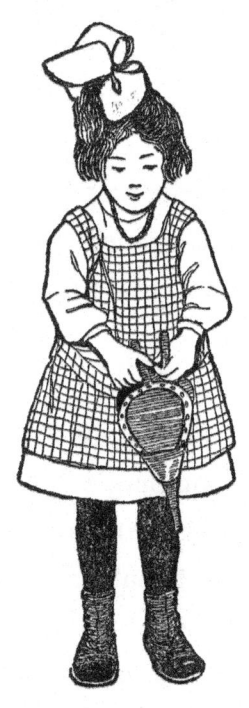

THE LUNGS ACT LIKE BELLOWS

It is because the little blood-boats float around and around—in a ring as it were, or in a circuit, that people are in the habit of saying that the blood circulates all through the body. They call this complete round made by the blood, the circulation.

When the little Dwarfs are both in a good temper, and work briskly, and when the little ships are all in good repair and nicely loaded, the master of the house knows that all is well; so he often says that his circulation is good, for he feels just warm enough, well and happy.

But when the little Pumping Dwarfs are in a bad temper, when they do not do their work well, or when the little ships are not properly cleaned, repaired and loaded, the master knows that something is wrong; he complains that his circulation is poor, that he feels too cold or too hot, and is sick and unhappy.

What Makes the Twins Cross

It may be that some of you wonder what can make the Twin Pumping Dwarfs cross. Well, I can tell you. They never object to hard work, and will plod on, provided the master sees to it that there is enough good food and air to load the boats. The Dwarfs are even ready to work faster every once in a while, if their master wishes to enjoy a little run.

But, if they have to keep on tugging at their ropes without getting any chance at all to snatch their wee rest between times, or if they are working so hard merely to send out half-laden blood-boats, they are very apt to get angry.

Sometimes they send telegrams up to the master saying: "Here! you had better be a little careful! It won't do to strain this delicate machinery. It can get out of order, you know; and if it gets badly out of order, neither you nor the wisest doctor who ever lived can get it right again! Don't you think you ought to give us a wee chance to rest? If you don't, we may strike and refuse to work at all. You know that if we do not send fresh blood to all your servants, and to all parts of your house, to keep it clean and in good repair, no work can be done in it. It will all go to pieces, and then you will have to move out whether you are ready to go or not!"

Or else they say: "Why don't you eat wholesome things and breathe plenty of nice fresh air? You know it is your business to do so, and that if you do not, the blood-boats cannot be properly loaded. Here we are working away night and day, sending them out only half loaded!

"They certainly are not carrying food and air enough to keep your servants in a good temper, neither are there building materials enough to keep your house in good repair, let alone to make it as big as it should be, to suit your wants. Can't you use a little common sense, and look after things a little better? After all, *you* will suffer most in the end if all does not go right, so do try and be sensible!"

The master should realize that what the Twin Servants say is perfectly true, and that as he can occupy the house only as long as their pumps are working nicely, he had better pay good attention to their warnings. If he is wise, therefore, he will see that there is enough good food and air to load all the blood-boats, and he will stop running, jumping, or overtaxing himself, whenever the Dwarfs call to his notice that their poor machinery is thumping too hard in its efforts to send the blood-boats along fast enough to do all the work he wishes.

How to Treat a Cut

The pipes leading to and from the heart, run under your skin in all directions. Most of the bigger pipes are so far inside that you cannot see them, but a few run near enough to the surface to enable you to trace their course. In all the pipes coming from the heart, you can generally feel, or hear, the thumping of the pump.

When a doctor wishes to know whether your Pumping Dwarfs are in a good temper, he always lays his fingers on a certain spot in your wrist. There he feels the blood run through a pipe, and he can count the strokes of the little pump.

He knows just how many times the Dwarfs should pull their ropes every minute, and by "feeling your pulse," as it is called, he finds out whether they are doing their duty. If the pulse beats too fast, he knows you have been overexerting yourself, or that you have a fever; if it beats too slowly, that the Dwarfs are cross because the blood-boats are not properly loaded, or because there is not liquid enough to fill the little rooms as often as they would like.

When you cut yourself, you can tell by the color, and especi-

How to Treat a Cut

ally by the way it flows, whether it is nice new blood which is streaming from the wound, or whether it is old, used-up blood. If the blood is on its way *from* the heart and is new, it will look bright red and will flow in jets or spurts, each coming with the tug which Dwarf Number One gives to his ropes.

In that case, you should hold the cut in such a way that the blood would have to run up hill to reach it from the heart. That will check the flow a trifle.

If it is a very deep cut, which bleeds hard, hold your hand or finger over the place so as to stop the blood from flowing. Then tie, or get some one

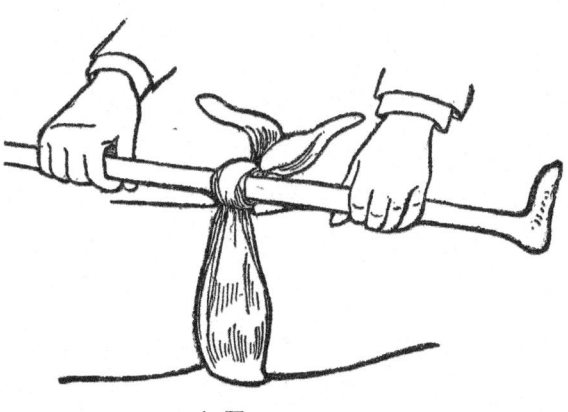

A TOURNIQUET

else to tie, a handkerchief, cord, or bandage very tightly over the cut. Next, run a pencil, or a bit of stick in this bandage, and turn it around and around in the way your mother or teacher will show you. Every turn you give the stick will serve to make the bandage tighter, and by and by, it will press so hard on the pipes under the skin, that it will stop the blood from flowing, until a clot can form, and act as a cork to stop up the hole.

If the blood flows in jets, it is always best to send for a doctor right away, so that he can bandage the wound properly.

But you must always try to stop the bleeding as I have explained, without waiting until he comes. You must not wait for the doctor to do it, because when the blood flows in jets it has to be checked at once, or the wounded person may bleed to death.

If the blood from any cut is dark red and flows evenly, you may be sure that it is worn out blood, on its way *back* to the heart. It does not matter so much therefore, if you do lose a little of that. To stop its flow you can tie a bandage in the same way as I described, and the blood will soon stop flowing. If it is a very big and deep cut, draw the two sides as closely together as you can before you tie it up, then send for the doctor so that he can sew it up.

Except in the case of very bad cuts or wounds, the blood on coming against the air, soon grows thick enough to form a clot which stops up the opening, prevents the loss of any more blood, and finally helps to heal the injured part, where all the little white boats now hurry with new building materials.

Any child who gets a bad fall or knock, can greatly lessen the pain, and prevent an ugly black-and-blue mark by wetting a folded cloth in hot water, and laying it on the spot. The water must be just as hot as one can bear it, and the cloth must be changed very often, so as to keep very hot water all the time on the hurt.

The heat brings the blood to this place, as you can easily see, for it gets very red. Then the little blood-boats all come rushing there in a hurry, laden with food and air, and they quickly

How to Treat a Cut 71

give up their loads. The white boats come too, and thus the damage is repaired as quickly as possible.

QUESTIONS.—What is your pumping station called? Can you explain where the Twin Dwarfs live, and how many rooms they have? Can they see each other and visit each other? What does Pumping Dwarf No. 1 do with the red blood which pours through the trap door and fills his upper room? When the lower room is full of blood, what does the dwarf do? Where does this squeezed out blood go? How does it travel all through the body? What are the blood boats; how are they loaded; where do they go, and what for? Blood boats going from the heart are loaded with repair material; what do those coming back to the heart bring? Who receives the returning boats, and how and where is the dirty blood cleaned? What makes the Twin Dwarfs angry? When you are cut and the blood comes out by jerks what should be done? How should you treat a bruise?

CHAPTER VI

How to Air Your House

WHEN we talked of the front door, in the beginning of this book, we said that air could easily come into the house through the mouth, and that there was an air-tube or stairway running down into the body just in front of the food tube or stairway. It is about this air, or windpipe, as it is also called, that you are going to learn to-day.

All houses need a great deal of nice fresh air. Ordinarily houses can be kept full of pure air, or well ventilated, as it is called, if all the windows are opened wide every morning, and if some of them are left partly open during the rest of the time in the rooms where people sit or sleep.

But your body needs fresh air every second almost. If you stopped breathing for more than a minute, you would feel very uncomfortable indeed, and if no new air at all came into your little house for about five minutes, you would have to move out, and all your body would surely die.

Because you need air while you are eating, it is not always possible to breathe through the mouth. A way was therefore provided so that you need never fall short of your air supply.

This way is through the nose. The nose is really the chimney of your little house. If all is well, the two nostrils,—air-passages, or pipes in your nose,—are always wide open. The air from outside rushes into these narrow passages, which open down into your throat.

The air on coming into these passages is warmed a little, and as it passes through the fine hairs growing inside the nostrils, all the bits of dust, and little shreds of cotton and down are caught fast, and not allowed to go down into the body. They are not wanted there, and would do much mischief, so the little hairs are always on guard to prevent their going down. The air also passes over wet cushions, all covered with fine skin; under this skin run many, many little nerves. They keep close watch over every breath of air that comes in, and telegraph up to the big central station, in the top of the head, reporting just how this air feels to them.

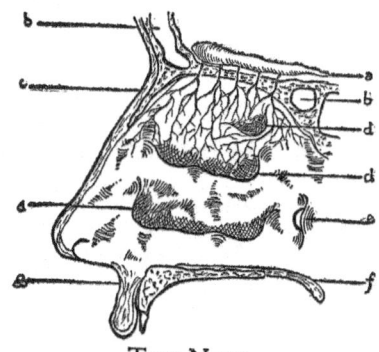

THE NOSE

a. Nerve of smell at the base of the brain. b. Air spaces in the skull bones. c. Branches of the nerves of smell. d. Curved curtains of bone. e. Opening of the tube to the ear. f. Soft palate. g. Upper jaw-bone.

Because these tiny nerves enable people to smell, they are very useful indeed. Any air which smells bad, is sure not to be good for the body. If the air smells fresh and clean, it is just right. Strongly perfumed air, even when we like the odor, is not good for us. Some people may be strong enough to bear it without great discomfort, but strong smells of any kind, are very likely to make babies or sickly people very ill.

About Choking

When the air has been sifted by the fine hairs, and tried by passing over the moist cushions in the nostrils, it is allowed to turn down into the back of the mouth and rush down the throat, or windpipe. That always stands wide open, except when food has to pass over it on its way to the food staircase.

Then, as you know, the little door keeper at the head of the windpipe shuts his trap-door, for nothing but air is wanted down in the windpipe.

Sometimes, when people talk or laugh while they are eating, or when they are not careful, both air and food try to get down-stairs at the same time. This always makes trouble, for if the little trap-door is not tightly closed when food passes over it, a few crumbs are likely to tumble down into the windpipe.

When this happens, there is a big fuss down there. The gatekeeper is frightened, for he knows that if any food gets down into the breathing room, the lungs or bellows of the body won't be able to use it or get rid of it, and that will make them so sore and uncomfortable that they may stop work entirely.

He therefore quickly sends a telegram down the windpipe, which is all lined with hundreds of little fans or whips. As soon as news is received that something is coming down which

About Choking 75

is not wanted there, all these little fans or whips begin to fan or whip upward.

The crumb or dust is therefore caught on its way downward, and fanned, or batted, up-stairs again. But all this causes such a to-do in the windpipe, that you hear a noise like coughing or choking. This is kept up, until the stray bit of food or dust has been driven right out of the windpipe again.

Very little children, who are too small to understand all that you have learned about the air and food pipes, often talk or laugh while they are eating. Then they choke. In their distress they generally double up and bend over forward while they are coughing. This is not best for them, because the straighter the windpipe is kept, the quicker the little fans or whips can bat the crumbs or dust out again.

Grown people, therefore, often point quickly up at the ceiling, saying: "Oh! Look at the little bird!" Most children are so eager to see a bird, that although they may be coughing very hard they quickly tip their heads back to look up.

This is the very best thing which can happen, for the crumb and dust can then fly right up, and the coughing stops. It is only when looking up won't answer, that one should slap a choking child on the back. Then, a pretty hard thump will help to drive the stuff up again, but as children do not understand why you slap them, this always seems rather an unkind way to end the trouble.

You may think that it is very wrong to say: "See the bird up there!" when you know perfectly well that there is no bird near the ceiling at all. But in a case like this, you are merely *fooling* the child for a minute for his own good. Most children too small to understand why you made them look up, will be quite satisfied if you say: "Oh, can't you see any bird? I don't see any either, so perhaps it has gone away."

When they are a little older, they will understand that it was not really a lie you told, and they will be glad to make use of this simple plan to save some other poor little tot from the pain which a bad choking fit often causes.

When I was too small to understand about the food pipe and the windpipe, my papa used to help me by making me look up for the little bird, and when I asked why I coughed so hard, he used to say in fun, if it had happened on a week day: "Perhaps it was because you made a mistake and tried to swallow down your Sunday throat!" If it happened on a Sunday, he always said: "Hello, why do you try to use your week day throat on Sunday?"

This always made me laugh and thus kept me from crying. But just as soon as I grew big enough to understand, I was told all about the pipes, and learned that the Sunday and week day throat story was only a bit of nice fun and nonsense.

The Speaking Dwarf

In the place in your throat where you can feel a lump, there is a kind of box. All across this box are stretched elastic cords,

The Speaking Dwarf

called muscles. We will make believe that a Speaking Dwarf lives in this box, and pulls these muscles apart to let the air in. Then he draws them more or less shut when the air comes out. If the master has nothing to say, the Dwarf leaves the muscles open, so that the air can pass in and out freely. But if the master wants to talk, the Dwarf quickly places the muscles in such a way that the air shakes them more or less hard.

Now those muscles are very like an elastic band, which you twang when it is tightly stretched. You know that such bands give forth different sounds, according to the way in which they are stretched. The Speaking Dwarf is so very clever, that he knows just exactly how to handle these muscles or bands, so as to give the kinds of sounds his master wishes.

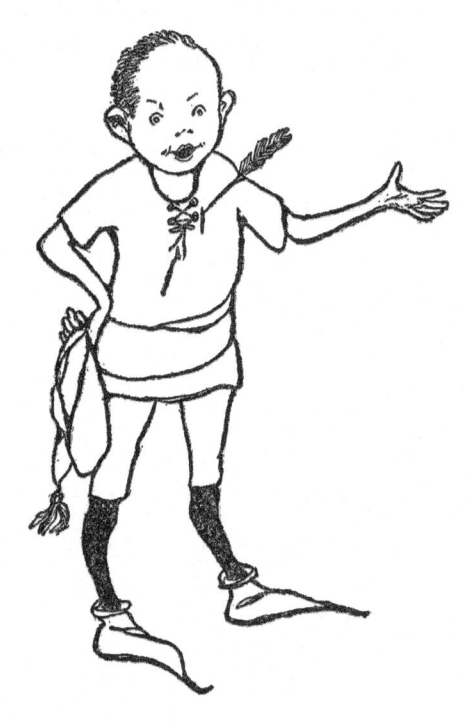

THE SPEAKING DWARF

If the air which comes down into the speaking-box is very cold or damp, it is bad for these delicate muscles. It often makes them so sore, that they get red and swollen. When such a thing happens, the Speaking Dwarf can no longer make them give out nice clear sounds, and then people often say: "How very hoarse that child is! Why, she must have a sore throat."

If you want to save trouble and stay well, you should always keep your mouth shut, and breathe only through your nose. Then, no dust, no food, and no damp or cold air can get down into your speaking-box, to make the muscles sore. But if you cannot breathe easily through your nose, you really ought to see a doctor; he will find out what is wrong and perhaps he can set it right.

After passing through the speaking-box, the air goes still further down the tube. Near the bone, which you can feel across the top of your chest, and which is called the collar-bone, this tube divides into two branches, both of which lead down into the lungs, which are fine bellows.

The lungs (or lights as the butcher calls them), are two big lumps of pink, sponge-like flesh. They fill up all the space inside the chest which is not taken up by the heart, or by the tubes which we have already talked about.

You have surely seen how a dry sponge can suck up water, and swell out bigger and bigger, the more water it holds. Well, the lungs act very much in the same manner, only *they* suck up air. When you draw as long a breath as you can, your lungs suck up so much air, and swell out so big, that your chest is not large enough to hold them, and has to widen out as far as it can.

Whenever your chest spreads out in that way, some bones, called ribs (which you can feel), rise up a little to give more room. A big band of muscle, which divides the chest into an upper and lower story, and stretches between the heart and lungs above, and the stomach and liver beneath, flattens out when you draw a long breath. Of course, that helps to make more space for the lungs; but, at the same time it crowds the stomach, liver and bowels further downward. Then, the skin over the abdomen, or belly, has to stretch a little so as to make room enough for them. If your clothes are as loose as they should be, you can easily feel your chest and sides swell out, whenever you draw in just as much air as you can hold.

If you want to have a fine broad chest, so that you can sing, speak, walk, and run, well and easily, it is a good plan to take as long breaths as you can, whenever you are sure the air is good and pure.

A person who breathes nothing but pure air, draws deep breaths as often as possible, and who never wears clothes tight enough to prevent the chest and sides from swelling out as much as they please, is sure to be very strong and well, unless something else is very wrong somewhere in his little house.

Where the Blood-Boats Get Their Air

The air, which rushes down into the lungs, fills every one of the little holes in them. All around these small holes there is a fine network of tiny little tubes. In these little tubes float the blood-boats all laden with bad air, and refuse. As they pass along they cleverly unload all the bad air, get rid of their refuse, and take good air in exchange.

They do this so very quickly and neatly, that by the time you cannot hold your breath any longer, all the boats then in the lungs are ready to sail back to the heart, from where they will begin a new journey. Then the band of muscle which had

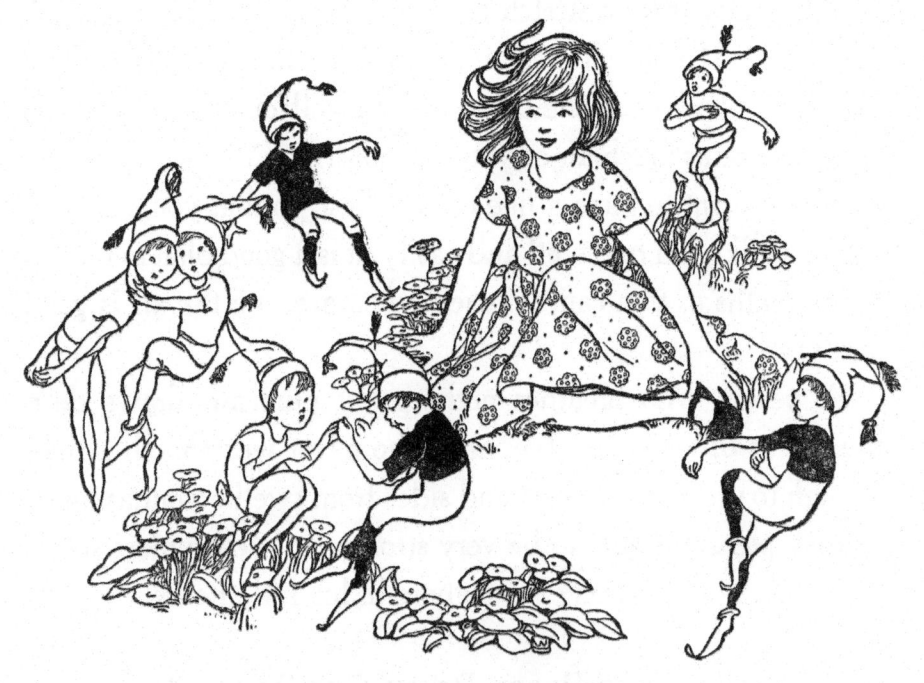

THE CHILD AND HER LOYAL SERVANTS

been forced down, springs back again, like an elastic when you let go of it, and as it rises and the ribs sink, the lungs are squeezed so that they can no longer hold all the air in them, and blow it up-stairs again.

As the lungs have given a large part of the *good* air to the little blood-boats, and taken *bad* air and refuse in exchange, they are very glad to get rid of it in this way.

When the bad air and the refuse is sent up the windpipe, all the little whips help to drive it out of the body through the mouth and nose. We know that this air is no longer good and fresh, because if you breathe into a bottle, in which a live mouse, or bird, or other small animal has been placed, the bad air soon makes them faint, and if they were left in it they would surely die.

All the air we breathe out contains a kind of gas which is bad for us, but which the plants suck up greedily as long as there is any light or sunshine. The plants, you know, are alive too, but while we breathe with our lungs only, they breathe all over, through wee openings in their stems and leaves. They not only eat up the air bad for us, but give out air good for us. In that way, all plants and animals—for men are animals you know—keep up an exchange as long as they live.

Doctors say that every time you take a good long breath, you take in about half a barrelful of good air. So, of course, every time you let it out again, you throw out half a barrelful of bad air.

Besides the gas which is bad for you, but good for plants, you throw out a little water every time you breathe, as you can see by breathing against a pane of glass or a mirror. The water you breathe out is like very fine steam. On a cold day you can *see* this vapor, but you never notice it when the air out of doors is nearly as warm as your breath.

You *cannot see* the bad gas at any time; you can see the refuse water only sometimes, and you cannot see the rest of the waste given off by the lungs, because it is much finer than the dust which you see dancing in a sunbeam. Still, you can *smell* the bad gas, and you can *feel* it. If you come from out of doors into a closed room where many people are sitting, you will notice right away how bad the air smells, and that it makes you pant and gasp just as if you had been running.

If you are sitting in a room where the air becomes bad, you may not notice it by the smell, but your cheeks will soon get red and hot, you will feel sleepy and stupid, and your head will ache. All this is because there is not fresh air enough in the room to keep your blood-boats nicely loaded, and because all the servants down below are grumbling hard, and giving you a headache, so as to call your attention to the fact that something is wrong.

You know that your Pumping Dwarfs cannot go and open a window, or run out of doors where there is plenty of air to be had! But if the master of the house is wise, he looks after his servants' comfort, by paying great attention to the kind of air he breathes. He also keeps a window open in his room at night, changes the air in the house often by opening both door and windows wide, and never stays in a place where he feels that the air is bad.

Some people, who do not know about the little blood-boats, the big bellows, and the Pumping Dwarfs, fancy that as long as you can breathe at all, everything is all right. They seldom open their windows, and were it not that fresh air *will* steal in through every crack in the doors, floors, windows and walls, and that it rushes up and down the chimneys, these foolish people would soon contrive to kill themselves.

As it is, they are not nearly as healthy, strong, or happy, as they would be if they had plenty of fresh air; neither can they study or work half as well, or enjoy their play as much. In fact, all doctors will tell you that bad air not only makes people feel badly, but makes them very cross, stupid and sometimes even wicked. They say that even little children are often fretful and naughty, merely because their poor little bodies do not get enough fresh air.

How Bad Air Kills

Once upon a time, during a war in India, one hundred and forty-six English prisoners were locked up in a place, so very small, that there was scarcely room enough for them to stand up in it. They were driven into this room at the sword's point and then the door was shut tight.

It is very hot in India, and as there were only two windows at one end of this room, the captives breathed up all the good air in a very few seconds. Then they began to pant and gasp, struggled to get near the windows, and tried to break down the strong door; but all in vain.

They were kept until morning in this awful place, which was known as the Black Hole. When the guards opened the door, all but twenty-three of the poor prisoners had died from

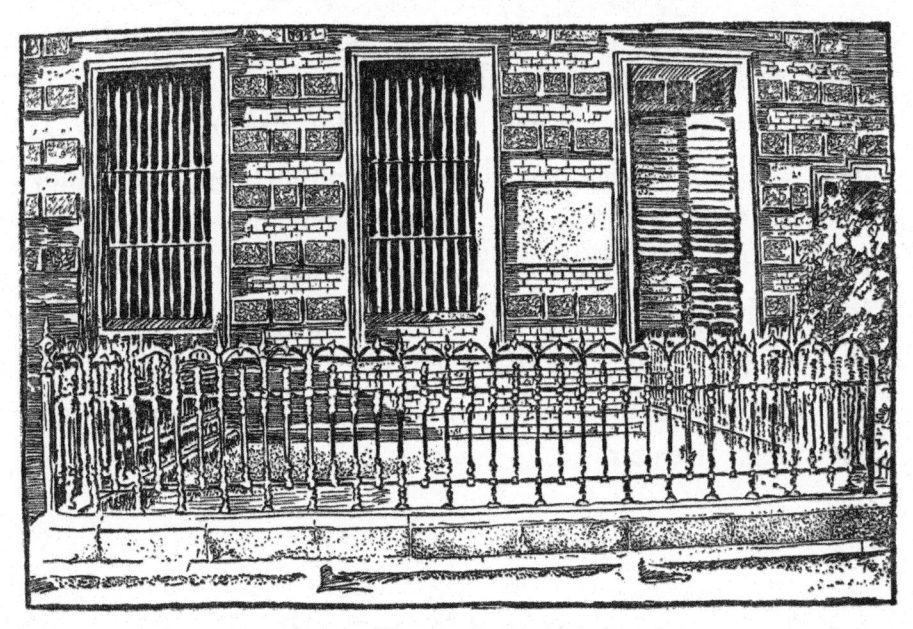

BLACK HOLE AT CALCUTTA

lack of air, and these twenty-three were so weak and ill that they never got perfectly well again.

You can see by this true story, how very dangerous it is to stay in places where the air cannot be changed often enough. Even if you do not die, like these poor prisoners, you are breathing bad air, the very air your lungs blew out as unfit for use.

How Bad Air Kills

You would rightly think it horrid if any one tried to *drink* dirty water or to *eat* swill, but it is just as nasty to *breathe* bad air, even though you cannot see how bad it looks.

Now there are many people in this world, who are very clean and particular about everything, except about the air they breathe. Some of these people are afraid to open the windows and change the air, because they say they catch cold so easily. But if they opened their windows often enough, and breathed nothing but fresh air, they would soon grow so much stronger that they would cease to catch cold so easily. They get sick, simply because the little blood-boats cannot get enough air to carry to all the different parts of the body so as to keep them in first-class order.

People who breathe the same air over and over again, are, besides, running the risk of catching some dreadful disease. For, with the air, the lungs blow out tiny seeds or germs of sickness. These are far too small to be seen, and if there were plenty of fresh air in the room, they would rise up to the ceiling, float out of the windows, be caught up by the wind, and carried high up in the air, where the hot sun would soon kill them.

If these germs cannot get out of the room, they are apt to be drawn into the lungs of any person who is not very well. There they are sure to grow, and to make that person very ill with scarlet fever, diphtheria, or whatever the disease may be. If the person does not catch the disease, it is only because the little

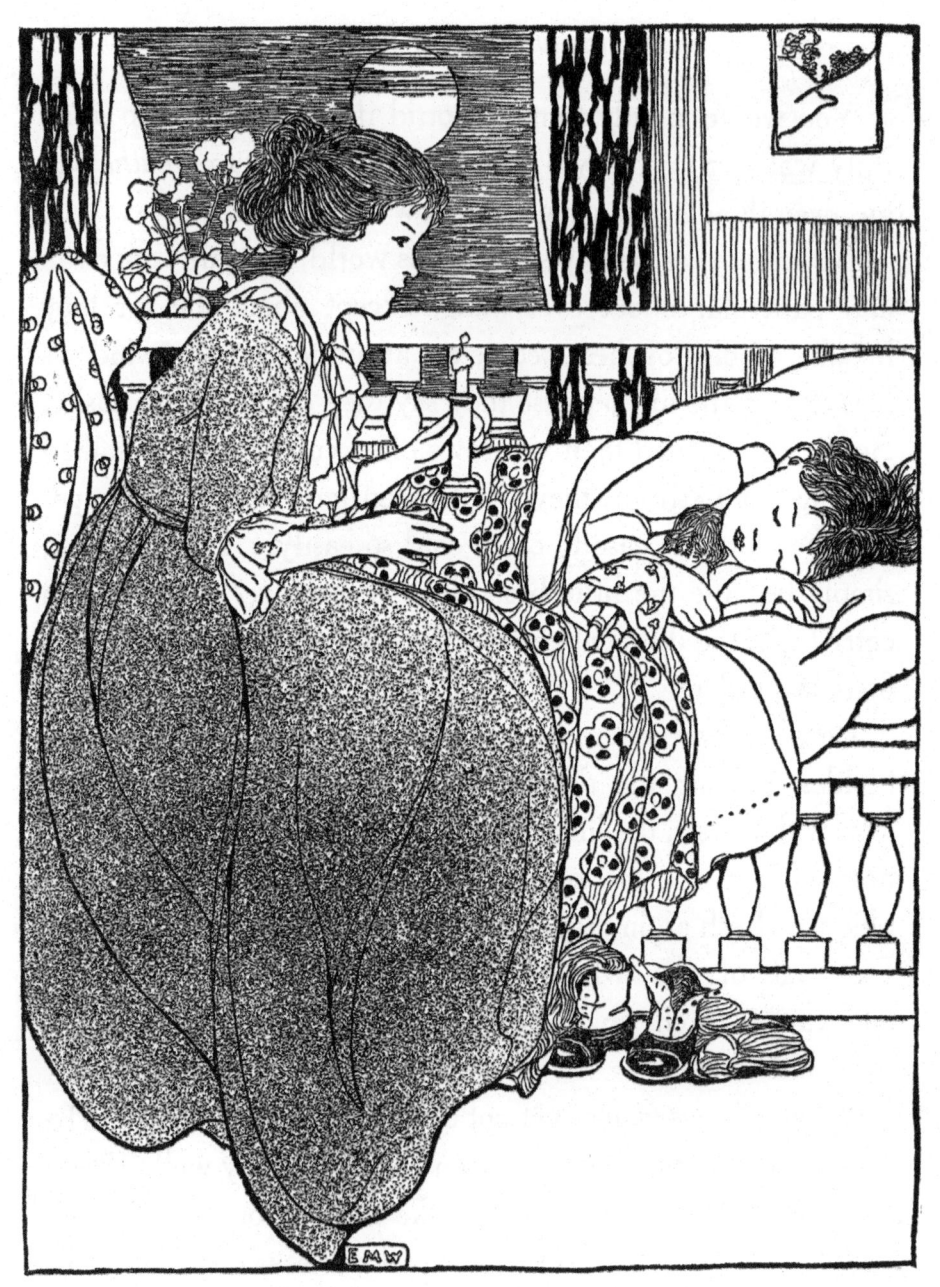

PLENTY OF FRESH AIR WHEN YOU SLEEP

How Bad Air Kills

blood-boats can still manage to carry enough good air to keep the body well.

The worst air in any room is always near the ceiling and near the floor, and the best in the space between. That is the reason why it is far wiser never to sleep on the floor or on too low a bed. But if you open your windows top and bottom, all the bad air in the room can escape, while fresh air takes its place.

Little babies suffer even more from bad air than older children, so if you want your little brothers and sisters to thrive, you should always be willing to take them out whenever mamma wishes. If they are out every nice sunny day, and if the room in which they play or sleep is always well aired, they will be rosy and happy, and will be much easier to manage.

Of course, babies catch cold very easily, and must therefore be carefully guarded from all draughts; but if the air they breathe is always pure, they are far less likely to take cold. Whenever it is too stormy to take baby out, you should carry him into another room while you open the windows wide.

If for any reason you have to stay in one room only, you can wrap baby up, just as if you were going to take him out, and then throw the windows and door wide open. In a few minutes the room will be well aired, and if you remove baby's wraps, little by little, after the windows are all closed, he will not be chilly, and you will both feel much brighter for the change of air.

Very few children, even among the rich, get air enough,

and still air is free to everybody, and does not cost a cent. The poorest person who ever lived can have all the air there is, if only willing to take the trouble to get it. If you live in a crowded city, it is not as easy to get fresh air as if you live out in the country. But even in the city, houses have doors and windows, and people can generally go up on the flat roofs. Besides, all who can walk, can go out into the parks, where good pure air can always be found.

THE NEED OF AIR

Sick people need a great deal of fresh air; the more they get, the quicker they are likely to be well again. Still, in some sicknesses, one has to be very careful not to let the *cold* air blow in upon the bed, although the patient must have *fresh* air all the time. To make sure of this, you can either open the window in the next room (keeping the door open between), or you can tack some thin cloth over an old fly screen, set it in the window frame, and open the window. The air can then sift slowly through the cloth, and you will thus secure enough without hurting even a sick person.

There was once a doctor, who had a dear little girl. She met with a terrible accident, which hurt her back so badly, that she had to sit still all the time. She could move her hands and arms a little, but was unable to go out to drive, or to be rolled around in a chair or carriage, because the least little jar made her suffer greatly.

Her father loved her very dearly, took the best care of her, and gave her everything that love or money could find to please her. She had a beautiful room, nurses who watched over her night and day, and the best food and medicine.

In spite of all this, the poor little maid grew thinner and thinner, and paler and paler, until her father's heart ached. One day he found her as white as a sheet, and so cross and hard to please that the nurse said with tears in her eyes: "What shall I do, sir, nothing suits her, nothing amuses her, and she cries nearly all the time!"

The father, almost in despair, said: "Poor little thing, it is because she has been shut up in the house so long. If she could only go out driving, it would be much better, for then she could have plenty of sun and air."

Looking out of the window while he spoke, the thought suddenly came to him that if his little daughter were carried out into the garden every day it might yet do her good.

So he had a nice little corner fixed up for her, and had her carried out there every fine day. At first, she stayed out only for a couple of hours, in the middle of the day; but when her father noticed that she always seemed more comfortable, and was less hard to amuse when out of doors than when in the house, he let her stay there all day long.

By the end of summer, the color had come back to her cheeks, and she was a very different little girl from the white-faced, peevish one I have told you about.

But her father was troubled whenever he thought of the

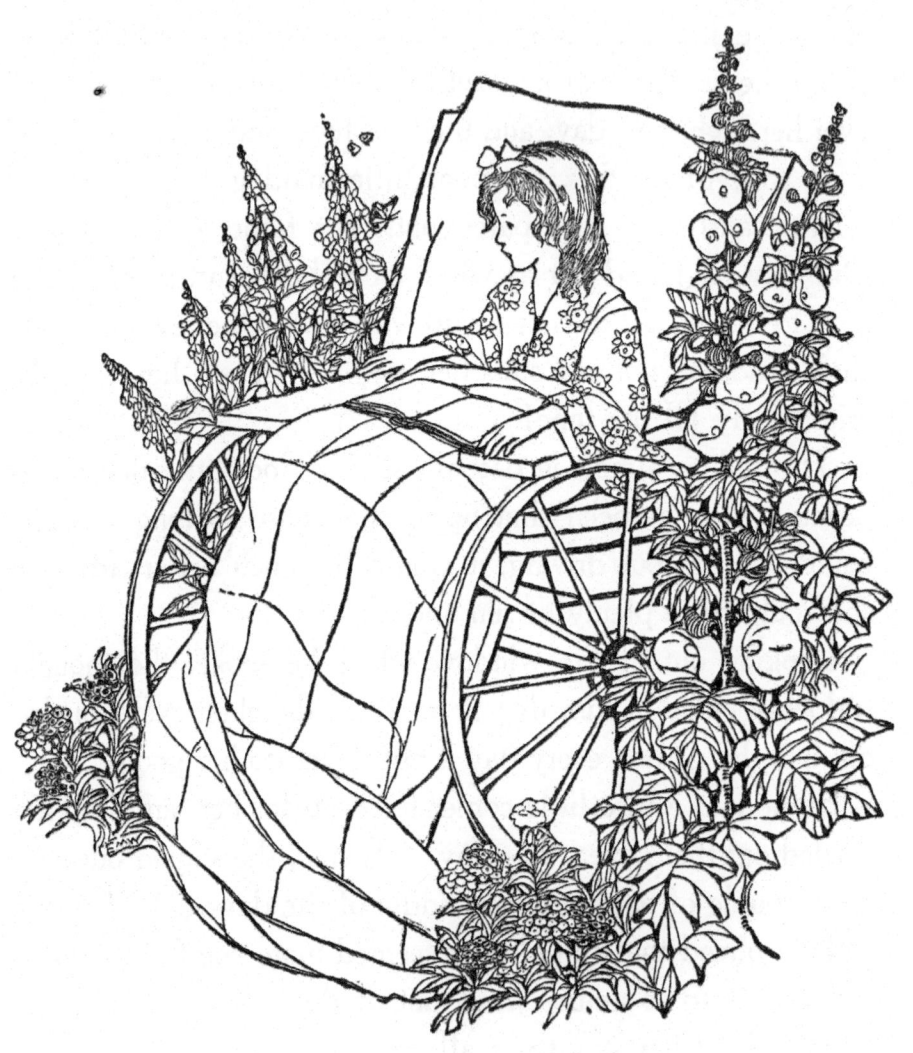

THE LITTLE INVALID IN THE GARDEN

coming winter. Finally he decided to try a new experiment. He had a nice fur coat and hood made for his little daughter;

The Need of Air

bought her fur mittens, and wrapped her up in thick fur rugs. Then bottles of hot water were tucked in here and there around her to keep her warm. Thus, she was able to sit out in the garden even on the coldest winter days.

With all her books and playthings around her, she was very happy out there, and as it was much too cold for her nurse to sit beside her, she told her to run into the house, and spent a good part of the time there alone, playing by herself. Of course, some one was always very near by, ready to come whenever she called, or rang her little silver bell, and her papa always stopped for a little chat with her on his way to and from his carriage, so that she should not feel lonely.

The doctor's neighbors, who had been away all summer, and who did not suppose that the poor child would ever be out again, were greatly surprised to see her lying out there in the garden when they looked out of their windows one day late in the fall.

They were surprised and greatly shocked when they noticed that she was all alone a good part of the time. Soon they began to say that it was dreadfully cruel to neglect a poor sick child in that way, and to leave her outdoors so late in the season. But every fine day the little maid was carried out there, and as it grew colder and colder, the neighbors became more and more indignant.

When the first snow began to fall, and no one came to carry her into the house, these neighbors could not stand it any longer, and one of them ran over to the doctor's office crying indignantly: "How can you treat that poor helpless child so cruelly?" The doctor gently asked her what she meant, and when she had explained, he smiled and said: "You saw my little daughter last winter, when we always kept her in a nice warm room and never let a breath of cold air blow upon her. Do you remember how pale and weak she was, how she cried and fretted, how poorly she slept, how little she ate, and how much trouble it was to amuse her or make her smile?"

"Yes, indeed!" said the woman, "and I admired your patience. I used to say you were the kindest father I had ever seen! And now, to think of your treating the poor little thing so, leaving her out there alone in the snow!"

"Well, come out there with me, and see whether you think I had better have her taken in," was all the answer the doctor gave her.

They went out together, and when the lady drew near enough to see the child plainly, she was amazed to perceive a laughing, rosy-cheeked, bright-eyed little face peep out from all those furs, and to hear a merry little voice cry out: "Oh, papa! It is too lovely for anything to be out in a snow-storm! Just look at all these pretty white stars clinging to my furs. A snowflake fell right into my mouth just a minute ago, and see, I have gathered nearly enough snow to make a ball to throw at you. You did not know I was going to snowball you, did you, papa?"

"No indeed, and if you do, perhaps I'll get some snow too, and wash your face," said her papa laughingly. "But aren't you cold, little daughter, and don't you want to come in?"

"Oh, no, papa, please, please let me stay out a little longer. It is such fun! Besides, this is nice dry snow, it cannot hurt me one bit, and I am just as warm as toast!"

A few minutes later the doctor took the lady back to his office, where he said: "Well, madam, do you really think I had better coop that child up in the house again, as I did last winter?"

"No, no indeed!" cried the lady. "Why, I never saw such a change in my life! And you say that the only medicine you have given her is plenty of fresh air and sunshine? I declare, I am going to try that medicine on my children too. I thought it was far too cold to let them go out, and I meant to keep them in all winter, because they are very delicate, but if a crippled child can sit outdoors all day, I guess a walk won't do them any harm!"

The lady went home to try the new remedy, and saw her little ones thrive like plants, for children too, need plenty of air and sunshine.

THE NEED OF SUNSHINE

In our last pages we said that if people, and children especially, wish to be well, they must get plenty of sunshine as well as plenty of fresh air. That reminds me of a funny story I once heard.

A wise doctor was once called to see a little girl who looked very pale and ill. She did not care to run about and play, and was so quiet and sad that her mamma was greatly troubled about her. After some time the doctor found out that the child was all right, but that her mother and nurse kept her bundled up so closely, and shaded so carefully, that the sun never had a chance to warm her skin.

He had preached fresh air and sunshine many a time, but the mother had not understood what he meant. She had sent her little daughter out of doors, but sunbonnets, veils and parasols, had kept every ray of sun away from the poor little thing.

There was a beautiful rose-bush in the garden which this little girl loved dearly, and the doctor,—who was "such a funny man"—suddenly proposed to dress that bush up in one of her suits of clothes.

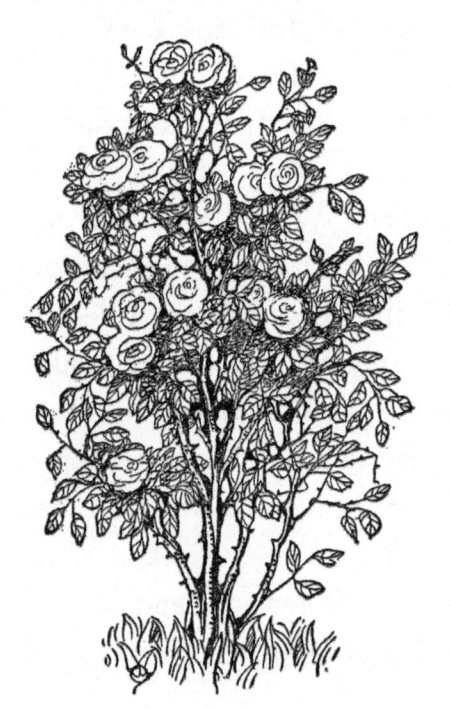

CHILDREN AND ROSES NEED SUNSHINE

The little girl thought this fine fun, although they had considerable trouble in getting all the garments on and around the poor rose-bush, which looked very queer all dressed up in its little mistress's garments! When they had finished, the doctor laughed and said: "Just let those things stay on the rose-bush until I come again."

A few days later, when the doctor and the little girl visited the rose-bush again, they found it withered and nearly dead. "Why! what does this mean?" said the doctor, making believe to be greatly surprised.

"It means that my poor rose-bush is dead!" cried the little girl. "Of course, the poor thing could not live without sunshine!"

"Neither can you," said the doctor. "You need sunshine too, or you will never be strong and happy. See, your rose-bush pined away after wearing all your clothes only a few days."

Both the little girl and her mother then understood what the doctor had been trying to tell them. After that the little girl was sent out of doors with no more wraps than other children, the sun was allowed to pour into the nursery where she played, and in summer, she ran along the beach barefooted and bareheaded, and took even more sun baths than dips into the sea. The result was that she was soon brown and rosy, full of fun and spirits, as hungry as a healthy child should be, and that she played all day and slept all night as hard as she could.

Sun and air are so good for everybody, that many sick people are now given sun and air baths so as to help them to get well. In fact, some people are kept out of doors nearly all the time, especially when they are troubled with weak lungs; and many a weak-lunged person has been quite cured by sleeping in a tent, and sitting out of doors all day long, in some place where the climate is both cold and dry. It is because sun and

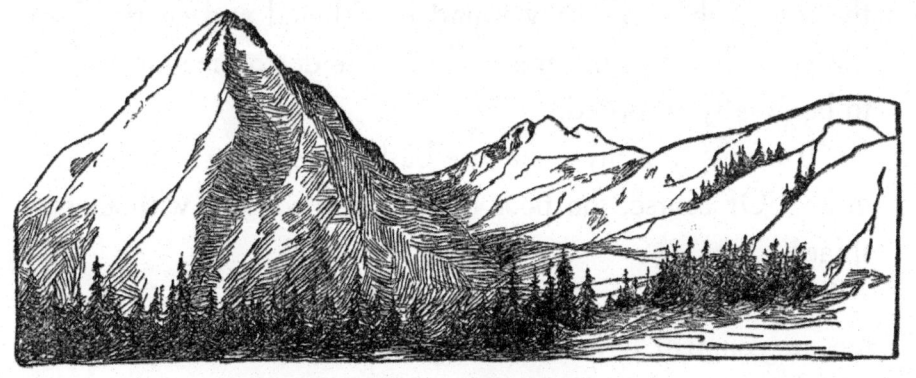

PURE DRY AIR AT THE MOUNTAINS

air are so good for such people, that doctors often send them to live in the Adirondack or other mountains, or out in Colorado, where cloudy days are very few.

QUESTIONS.—Since the Pumping Dwarfs need plenty of air to keep your blood clean, how can you get enough in your house? Where is the air, or wind pipe? Is it best to breathe through your mouth or your nose, and why? Should a crumb get into your windpipe by accident, what happens? Where does the Speaking Dwarf live and what makes him hoarse? When the air has passed Speaking Dwarf's box, where does it go? What fills all the little holes in the lungs like water fills a sponge? When your lungs are just as full as they can hold of air, how do chest, ribs, and muscle band act? Why are blood-boats waiting at every little hole in the lungs? Where does their load of bad air go? Is bad air a poison for men, animals and plants? Can very bad air kill, and should one ever breathe it unnecessarily? Where is the worst air in a room? Can you tell the stories that show how plenty of air and sunshine are good for even sick children?

CHAPTER VII

THE FRAMEWORK OF YOUR HOUSE

EVERY house has some kind of a frame, although you often cannot see it after the house is all finished. There is also a frame to your body, which you can *feel,* although it is all covered over so that you cannot see it.

As you know, the framework of a house is made of wood or iron beams; but your framework is all made of bone. If all the skin and flesh which cover and hide your bones were taken away, there would be nothing but the bone frame, or skeleton, left.

Every one has a bone frame to keep the soft parts of his body in good shape, and to protect the delicate parts. If you look at the picture of a skeleton, you will see that the skull is a kind of a bone box, made to hold the brain. The chest is a bone cage, made to protect your heart and lungs; and there is a sort of bone basin, made on purpose to hold the bowels, etc.

If we mention the backbone,—which is really a string of little bones, fitted nicely together,—the bones of the legs and arms, and of the hands and feet, we have spoken of all the principal beams in our bodies.

Still there are many different bones, and if you come to count them all separately, little and big, you will find about two hundred. Each of these bones has its own name, its own place, and its own use. Doctors know just where these bones are, what they do, and how to mend them when they are broken or out of joint. Besides, they know just what makes good and bad bones, and if called in time, they can often straighten crooked bones, and make sick bones well.

Even when you were a wee baby, so small and so soft that one hardly dared to touch you, all your bones were there. But they were not big and strong and hard as they are now. They were very small, and so soft that they could easily bend.

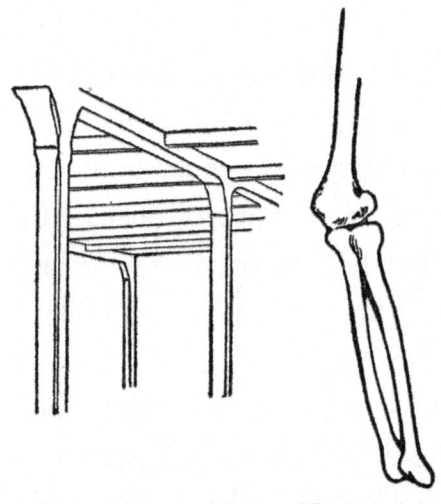

THE FRAMEWORK OF A HOUSE AND OF YOUR FORE-ARM

Bones keep growing bigger and harder, longer and stronger, from babyhood until you are about twenty-five years old. It is only then, that the framework of human houses is really finished, and that they cease to grow. Still, as long as we live, our bones are alive, and need the air and food which the blood-boats bring them night and day.

Bones are made of a tough animal material which can bend

easily. In the wee open spaces between this material, there are stored away the mineral parts, which make bones hard and brittle. We know that bones are thus queerly made, and you can prove it for yourself, if you choose to make the following experiments.

Take a chicken, or any other kind of a bone, put it in the fire and let it stay there about three hours, or until all the fat, or animal part, is burned up. Then take it out of the fire, very gently and carefully, and you will see that it looks much the same, but is all full of little holes. If you strike this bone with a hammer, it will fall into dust, for now that the animal part is burned away, there is nothing left to hold the mineral parts in place.

Now, take another bone, soak it three days in muriatic acid. Then, all the mineral part of this bone will be eaten up by the acid, and nothing but the animal part left. A bone which has been treated in this way, can easily be bent in any shape you please. It is so supple, that you can even tie it in a knot, but you cannot break it, because it is still very tough, although it has ceased to be brittle.

BABY'S BONES

Because soft bones can so easily be bent, we ought to be very careful to keep our bones straight as long as they are soft. That is one reason why babies must be handled with so much care.

All their bones are so very soft and tender, that they can readily be bent out of the right shape.

It is because a baby's bones bend so easily, that it is never wise to let him stand too soon. But some grown people are very foolish, and keep coaxing baby to stand, long before his poor little legs are really strong enough to bear his weight. Thus, his soft bones are bent a little, and baby grows up bow-legged.

Babies who are strong and light, can often stand and walk without hurting themselves when they are only nine or ten months old. But a weak, fat, or heavy baby, should not be expected or encouraged to walk until very much later. In fact, it is very much better for most babies not to try to walk until they are a year and a half old, for until then their bones are often not strong enough to hold them up without bending a little.

Baby will *want* to stand and walk just as soon as he feels

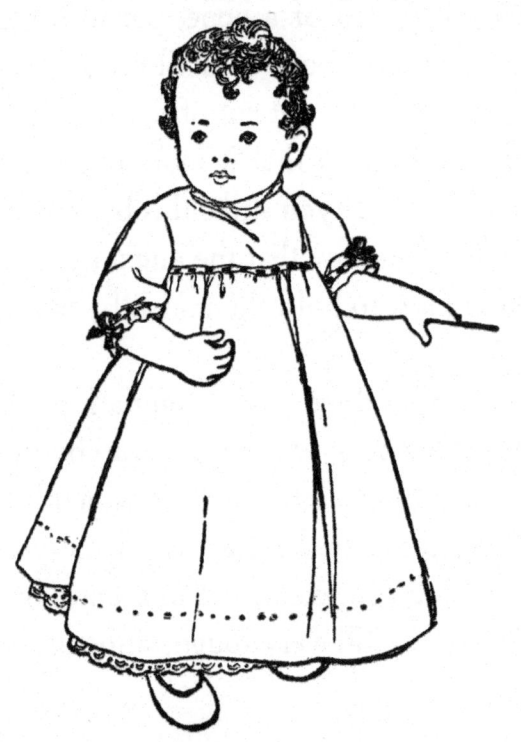

LEARNING TO WALK

Baby's Bones

strong enough to do so. Therefore, you must not coax or urge him, until he is quite ready. It is also because a baby's bones are soft, and bend easily without breaking, that you seldom hear of broken bones among very little children.

Although, as you know, the wee tots are always falling, they seldom get badly hurt. Still, one should never drop a baby, or bump his head because lifelong injuries are the result of such accidents.

The bones forming baby's head are not only very soft, but they do not join together, until he is nearly three years old. It is because the bones are not joined at first, that baby has a "soft spot" on the top of his little head.

You have surely been told to be careful always to touch that spot very, very gently. In that place, baby's tender little brain is not protected by any bone. A blow or knock there, or even a rough touch, might hurt the baby's brain so badly, that he might become very ill, or be an idiot all his days. You see now, why your mamma is so very gentle with the baby, and why she guards that "soft spot" with such loving care.

Young bones can so easily take a wrong shape, that mothers and teachers have to keep very close watch over the children to prevent their growing up crooked. Now, many children think it is just fussiness when older people keep reminding them to sit up straight, to stand on both feet, to hold their heads up, to throw their shoulders back, and not to twist their feet around chair legs.

But, mothers and teachers know that if you sit a few hours every day, with one arm on the desk and the other in your lap, your poor backbone will be all twisted. If it gets in the habit of twisting in this way, it will soon stay so, and then you will be deformed when you grow up.

There are some people in the world who are deformed and cannot help it. Some of them were born so, with others it is the result of some accident, or of some disease. But a child who grows up crooked, simply because he is careless, or who wilfully bends his nice straight bones into wrong shapes, is acting in a very wrong way, and will be very sorry later on.

How to Keep Straight Bones

In early childhood, the bones are so soft that they can bend almost any way we please. By ten, most children have the habit of sitting or standing in certain ways. If these habits are good, their bones are growing straight. But if the habits are bad, their bones are already a little crooked, and will go on growing more and more so, every day the wrong habits are kept up.

Every child who reads this book ought to stop and think whether he generally sits, and stands, and moves as he should. Does your mother or teacher have to tell you, many times a day, "Stand up straight," "Sit up in your chair," "Don't loll about," etc., etc.? If you hear these words often, you may be sure you are not treating your bones as you should.

I have seen careful mothers who were always reminding their children to hold themselves properly. These mothers thought of the future, and were anxious to have their children grow up with strong, straight frameworks for their bodies. But I have seen those very children obey in a half-hearted way, and sink back into the wrong position just as soon as mother's back was turned.

Some children, when reminded of this matter often get very cross indeed, and say or think: "Oh, dear, I do wish mother would let me alone! She does worry so about how I stand or sit. I *like* to sit crooked. What difference does it make to her? I don't care how I look."

No, you may not care one bit now, but when it is too late, when your bones have grown quite crooked, and when nothing can straighten them again, you will wish you had acted very differently, and you will say: "Oh! why didn't they *make* me do it whether I wanted to or not?"

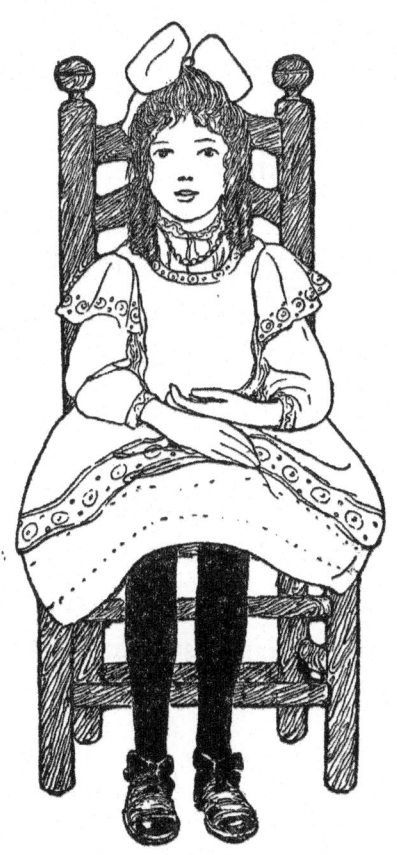

LEARN TO SIT PROPERLY

Now, if parents and teachers could give all their time to this one thing only, they might be able to *make* the children sit and stand correctly nearly all the time; but then, you see, they would have no chance to do anything else! How much wiser it would be, therefore, if every little house owner made up his mind, right now, to watch over this matter himself, and to see that his beams have no chance to be anything but straight and strong in the end.

The master in your house can easily look after the framework all the time, if he only chooses to do so. He can send telegrams all over the building, and his servants will be sure to obey any orders they receive. Then, every one will say: "See, so-and-so has a fine, graceful figure! Just look what a straight back he has! See how well he carries himself, and how easily he moves. He is a finely built fellow!"

This is much more pleasant than to hear some one remark: "Did you ever see such a crooked person as so-and-so? He moves about in such an awkward way, that I cannot bear to look at him!"

The Crooked Tree

There is a very old proverb which says: "As the twig is bent, the tree is inclined." This proverb is very true, as the following story will show you. In an orchard there was once a very crooked tree; so crooked, that instead of growing straight up into the air like all the rest, it bent far over until its trunk was almost lying along the ground.

One day, when the farmer and his son were in the orchard together, the boy noticed that crooked tree and asked his father why he did not cut it down.

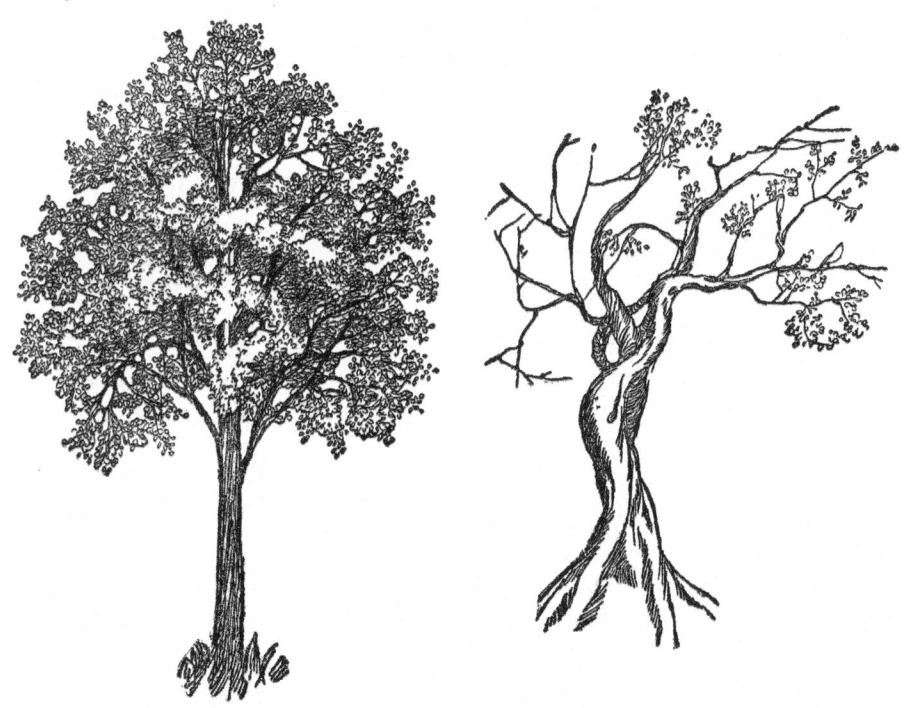

STRAIGHT AND CROOKED TREES

"Oh, I don't want to do that," said the farmer, "for it bears such fine apples!"

"Well, then, father, you really ought to straighten it, for it spoils the looks of this nice orchard!" answered the son.

"Yes," said the farmer, "it is a pity to have such a crooked tree in this orchard. You are quite right, my son, we must straighten it up."

So he sent for a man with a team of strong horses and bade him bring along chains and ropes. But after trying a long time, and all in vain, the man said: "It is no use, sir! That tree can never be straightened again. It has grown crooked. If you wanted a straight tree, you should have seen to it some years ago, when it was young. Then, a child could easily have bent it this way or that. Now, all the teams in the world could not pull it straight!"

This man was quite right, you see, and the proverb is right too. If you want young trees to grow up straight, you must watch them, and when they show any signs of leaning over, tie them to stout stakes. Those will hold them up until they have grown strong and upright. That is the way to have nice trees!

Now, boys and girls are very much like young trees, only as they do not keep still, they cannot be tied to stakes. But if boys and girls watch themselves, train themselves to sit up straight, always stand on both feet, hold their shoulders back, their knees straight, and their heads up, their bones will be sure to grow in the right way.

So, boys and girls, help your parents and teachers all you can, instead of hindering them as you do, and remember that it is not "nagging," but great kindness, when some one reminds you that you are not holding yourself properly.

You should also help your younger brothers and sisters to

keep their bones in the right shape, and bear in mind at all times how very careful you should be with the baby's bones, because they are the most tender of all.

Some of you may have had very bad habits until now, but you can change them, for it is not yet too late. Most of your bones grow until you are twenty, so, many of them can still be straightened out, even if they are a little out of shape when you are ten or twelve years old. But you will doubtless find that it takes a great deal of hard trying every day, and all day, to get rid of bad habits and to form good ones. Still, when good habits are formed, and the bad ones are quite forgotten, you will be able to trust your servants to keep them up, for they will do whatever you really wish.

It is the duty of every boy or girl to see that his or her framework is just as good and straight as it can be made. When you grow up, you will be very glad to have strong, good-looking houses rather than tumble-down shanties. In fact, some bodies are so fine and strong and well-cared for, that they deserve to be called temples, while others are so neglected, crooked, and ugly, that they no longer look like God's handiwork at all.

How to Have Good Bones

Most of our bones are hollow. That is what makes them light and strong at the same time. In the hollow there is some fat, called marrow, in and through which run many little veins, along which the blood-boats travel night and day.

All the bones of the body are made to fit nicely together. The place where two or more bones join together is called a joint. You all can surely point to your finger, elbow, and knee-joints, can you not? If a bone slips out of the place where it belongs, we say it is "out of joint."

Whenever this happens, it always causes pain. The best thing to do then is to keep perfectly quiet until the doctor comes. If the hurt is very bad, and is in your hand or foot, you can hold it in a basin of hot water. If elsewhere, put cloths dipped in hot water upon the aching part, and keep changing them often. This will lessen the pain, will prevent swelling, and the heat will quickly bring the blood-boats there to repair any damages.

If a fall or blow results in a broken bone, you should also keep very still until the doctor comes. But if the accident happens out of doors, when the weather is too cold for you to stay quiet, those who are with you should help, or carry you home, holding the broken parts firmly together, to prevent the bones from slipping any further out of place, or from running through the skin.

Hot water on a broken bone is also the easiest remedy until the doctor comes; but you should send for him right away, for the sooner the bone is set, the sooner the blood-boats can set to work to mend it by bringing new materials.

Broken bones generally grow together again in a month or six weeks, and if one keeps quite still, and minds all the doctor's orders, they will be just as good as new. Any neglect of the doctor's orders, or using a broken limb too soon, is sure to prevent the bone from healing properly.

When a bone does not heal aright, the limb proves more or less useless, and sometimes doctors have to break the same bone over again to get it straight and well once more. As this is even more painful than the first break, it is far wiser to see that the bone has a good chance to heal properly the first time it is damaged.

Plenty of bread, oatmeal, and wholesome food in general, is good for your bones; but too many sweets and too much soda water is very bad indeed for them. A child who drinks much soda water is very apt to have brittle bones and poor teeth. A tumble, which would only mean a bump or a bruise for some one else, may result in one or more breaks with a child who drinks much soda water. And these breaks will not heal as fast nor as perfectly, as if the child had never been allowed to drink soda water, save once in a very great while, as a special treat.

QUESTIONS.—Of what is the framework of your little house made? What is your bone framework called, and how do you know it is there? Touch your three bone cages and tell what they hold. About how many bones have you, and what is your backbone? Were your bones always hard? Why must you be very careful how you touch a wee baby? If you sit and stand badly, what will it do to your bones? Can a tree which has grown up crooked be straightened? How do the blood-boats travel up and down the bones? What do you call the place where bones join together? What can boys and girls do to secure a good frame. Why do parents and teachers often tell you to sit or stand differently? What should be done if a bone is out of joint? What should you do if you have a broken bone?

CHAPTER VIII

YOUR PULLEYS AND ROPES

WE have said that the bones or frames of our bodies are all covered with flesh, which lies like a kind of cushion around and over them. It is the flesh which gives our body its soft, rounded appearance.

The flesh which covers our bones is all made up of muscle and fat, through which run many of the pipes and blood vessels.

We have already learned about the blood vessels and the blood-boats, so we know how useful they are. The fat which is tucked away in the different parts of the body is also useful. It is made mostly from sugar, and it is stored up, so that the blood-boats can go and get it and use it, whenever anything happens to the stomach, bowels, or liver, so that they cannot send fresh supplies of food.

The muscles (what we call lean meat in beef, mutton, or any other kind of meat which comes on our tables) are very useful indeed. They are really the ropes by means of which the master pulls the bones here and there to make the body move. These muscles are fine and very elastic, and there are so many of them that they form bunches. The muscles bind all the bones together and keep them in place. If they were not so strong and so elastic, our body framework would

How Muscles Change Shape

wobble and fall apart like a badly jointed doll, or we would be stiff and immovable, so that we would look more like wooden statues than like graceful, active, living beings.

Besides being something like a house, our body can also be compared to a machine. In the latter case the muscles are the ropes and straps, which can be tightened or loosened, just as the owner of the machine pleases. The muscles not only cover all the bone framework of the body, but they form part of all the pipes, and the room walls and linings. They are everywhere, and everywhere they are useful, as you are going to see.

How Muscles Change Shape

All our muscles are very elastic and ready to obey the least message brought by the nerve telegraph, which runs all through our bodies in every direction. The muscles are so elastic, that they can also change their shape in an instant, and stretch out until they are long and thin, or tighten up until they are very short and thick.

If you wish to know just how your muscles act, lay your left hand on the upper inner part of your right arm. Now clench your right fist and draw it up towards your shoulder. As you do this, you can feel the tightening of the big muscle between the shoulder and elbow, can you not? In fact, it grows so thick and makes such a bump, that you can see as well as feel it.

People who use their muscles a great deal, have much larger and stronger muscles than those who sit still and do nothing. A boy who plays baseball, does gymnastics, rows and swims, or one who works on a farm or at some trade, has far more muscle (as it is called), than one who spends most of his time lolling in an easy chair, asking: "What shall I do?" or crying: "I don't know what to play next."

Girls who run, and jump, and play tag, who help mother in the kitchen and house-work, and who take care of the baby, also have more and better muscle than those who never do anything active or useful.

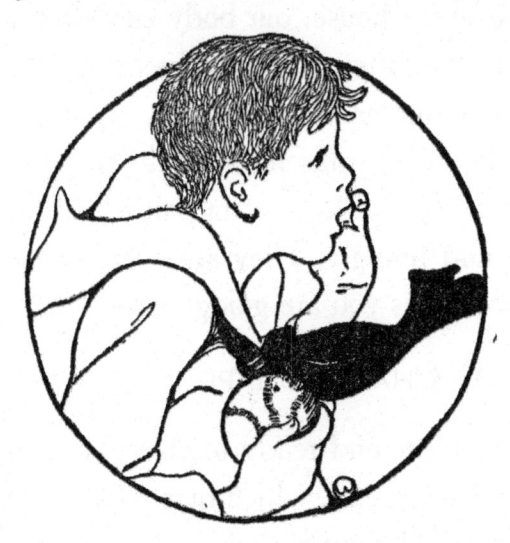

BASEBALL DEVELOPS MUSCLE

A child who is very active, who runs about a great deal, and who is never quiet save when asleep, keeps many of its muscles at work all the time. Every time a muscle moves, it uses up a little air and food, and wears out a little of its material. When muscles are very busy they use up more food and air than when they move quietly or are at rest.

For that reason, as soon as you begin to move them, the Pumping Dwarfs send the blood-boats out a little faster, for they know that the muscles need plenty of food and repairing stuff. The muscles are all fed and kept in good repair by these little blood-boats, which, besides food and building materials, bring all the air needed.

The muscles are very glad to get this food and air and new building materials to take the place of those which are worn out. Besides, the muscles have to get rid of the bad air, the waste food, and the worn-out materials, which those same little blood-boats carry swiftly away.

How to Treat the Muscles

If the muscles move so fast that they use up more food and air than the blood-boats can bring, even when the Pumping Dwarfs are sending them out as fast as they can, they soon feel very faint and weak.

Then they telegraph up to the master: "Can't you let us rest? We are tired. Stop a minute so we can get food and air enough, and so we can replace our worn-out material!" If the master minds this message, and makes the body rest, the muscles make up their loss, and they soon feel all right again.

But if the master pays no heed to the message, and keeps the muscles working, they get more and more tired, until they feel so faint they can scarcely do what he wishes. When this happens, they sometimes get cross and jerk. At other times they are sad and discouraged, and go on in a half-hearted way until they ache so hard that the master finds it out. Then,—as the ache disturbs him,—he generally sends word to them to stop moving.

Even while the master is sound asleep, the muscles are still at work. They are busy taking in food and air from the blood-boats, and getting new materials to repair the damages done by moving too fast and too long.

If they can get food and air enough while the master is asleep, and if they can get rid of all the waste, get new stuff, and enjoy a wee rest, they will be quite ready for a new day's work when the master awakes.

But if the master has not been careful to eat enough good food, or to drink enough pure water, and if he does not breathe enough fresh air, even while he sleeps, the blood-boats cannot carry enough supplies to the muscles. Then the muscles cannot repair damages, and when the master wakes up, and wants them to go to work, they are not in good condition to do so.

Then the master receives a telegram from them saying: "We don't feel like working. We are still aching hard. Leave us alone!" Some masters pay no attention to such messages as this, and make the poor tired muscles work on. Others say: "Very well, we'll both rest," and then they spend their time eating trash, or breathing bad air. This kind of rest does tired muscles no good at all.

But a wise master thinks: "Poor little muscles. I did not treat them fairly. They always served me well when I gave them food, air and rest enough. I must have stinted them in some way. Let's see, what did I do that was wrong? I stopped when they sent word they ached, and went to sleep, for I knew that the Pumping Dwarfs would send the blood-boats to them with food and air. Yesterday I ate plenty of good plain food, so surely the blood-boats had enough food to carry. Ah! I remember now what was wrong! I forgot to open my bedroom window last night!

"While asleep I breathed the same air over and over again, all night long. Of course the blood-boats could not get fresh air enough to carry to my tired muscles. That is why they are still cross and tired this morning. I am not a good master. I must be more careful. Now, I will go out of doors and take long full breaths, so as to send as much air as I can to those poor muscles."

A master who thus finds out just why his muscles are cross, and who honestly tries to supply what they need, will generally find that they are quite willing and ready to go to work again as soon as they have secured what they needed so badly.

The more exercise you take,—out of doors especially, where you are sure of having plenty of nice fresh air all the time,—the better it is for your muscles. For, when you exercise, you wear out the old muscle, and the blood boats bring materials to make new. With plenty of food, air, and the right materials, good new muscle is made, and every one knows how much better fresh, new things are than those which are old and worn out!

That is why parents and teachers urge children to run and play out of doors whenever they can, and that is why you should have plenty of exercise. Children of all ages need exercise, and so do the older people, only they often need less because you see their muscles are already full grown.

How to Train the Muscles

When muscles have enough food, air, and rest, they are apt to be quite healthy. But muscles need plenty of exercise as well as plenty of rest. If you wish your muscles to obey you quickly, and to do exactly what you wish, in the neatest and nicest way, you must first teach them how to do it.

The muscles are all willing servants of the master of the house, but he has to train them. If he trains them well, they will do his work well; but if he is careless and lets them do their work in any way they please, it will often be very poorly done.

You know how it always is. Good masters make good servants. In some houses everything is done neatly, the meals ready on time, well cooked, and all runs smoothly. Then we say: "So-and-so is a fine housekeeper and has beautifully trained servants. Everything runs as smoothly as clock work in that house!"

In other places, you find everything at sixes and sevens, the meals are not on time, the food is badly cooked, the rooms are untidy, and people rightly say: "So-and-so is a very poor housekeeper. Her servants are lazy and untidy and run the house any way they please. It is very uncomfortable there."

Now, since each one of us can train his muscle servants either to be neat, quick, and capable, or to be slow, lazy and un-

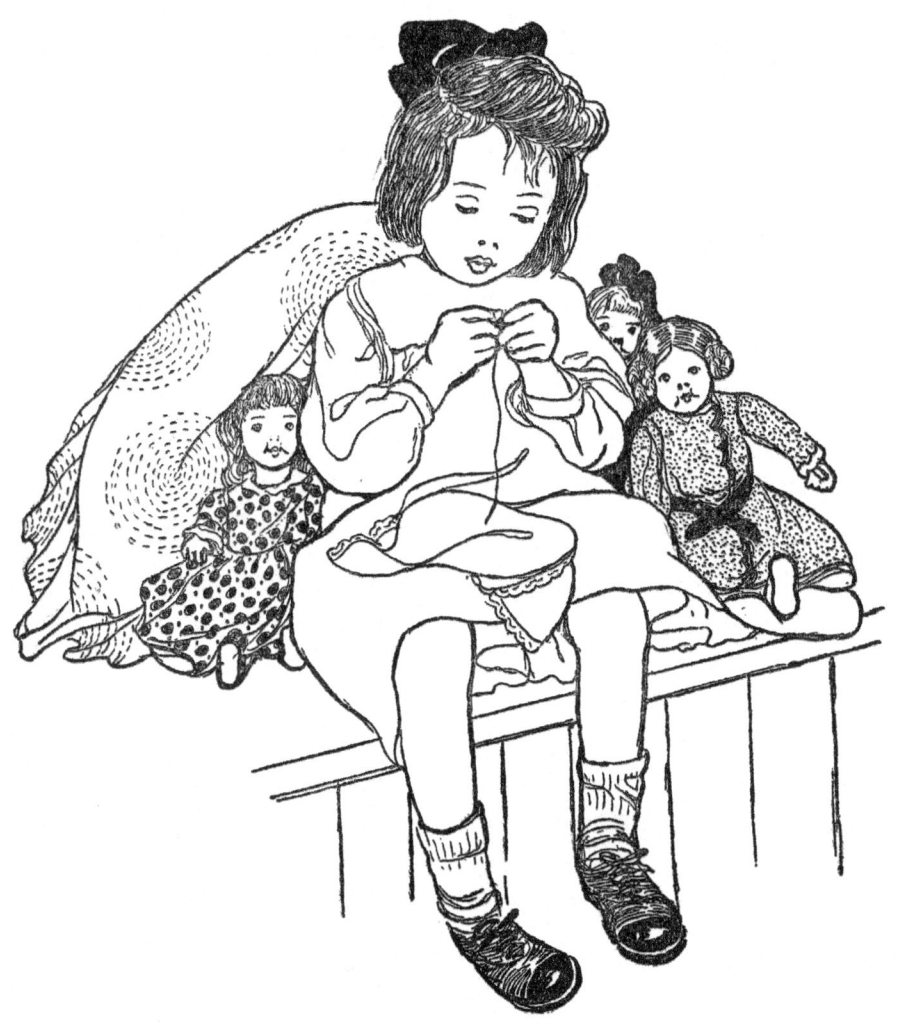

THREADING A NEEDLE

tidy, don't you think it is wisest to begin right away and make them really good servants?

You know how it is about such a simple matter as throwing a ball. A boy who knows just how to do it, picks up the ball, gives it a toss, and the ball goes just where he wishes. That is because he has practiced throwing balls until he is a fine pitcher.

A girl who has not practiced baseball playing does it in a clumsy way. The ball goes only a little distance, or strikes far from the spot where she wished it to go. But a girl can take a needle and thread it, neatly and quickly, while a boy in trying to do so acts "as if his fingers were all thumbs."

In both of these cases the muscles which have done the work often, and which have been trained to do it neatly, quickly, and without any fuss, are good servants, while those which have not been trained cannot do the work well. Girls can learn to throw balls just as well as boys, and boys can learn to thread needles just as well as girls, if they only choose to do so. But it takes practice to do either thing well.

If you allow your muscles to get into lazy, roundabout, awkward ways of doing things, you will have a great deal of trouble breaking them of these bad habits. But, still, you can do it, for every one who is not an idiot or a cripple, can train his muscles to do his work well.

With Brains, Sir

One day, an artist went into a fellow-painter's studio and greatly admired a beautiful picture he had just finished. The figures were so lifelike, and the colors so bright, that the visitor imagined there must be a secret way of preparing them and eagerly said: "I'd like to get my colors to glow like that. With what do you mix yours?"

"With brains, sir!" answered the painter, angry at being asked such a silly question.

Now I am going to tell you a great secret. That is that everything we do should be mixed with brains! There is a right and a wrong way of doing everything. Of course, every child who reads this, learned to dress himself or herself long ago. You dress yourselves every morning, do you not? Many of you even have to dress several times a day.

Each time you dress, you call your muscle servants and set them to work. Some children have trained their muscle servants so that they do that work neatly and quickly. The master up in their brain watches these servants closely, to see that they do their work properly. He always directs the hands, for instance, to seize and hold the stockings in such a way that they can be pulled on straight, and without needing to be twisted and turned to get the toes in the right place or the seam running up the back of the leg.

Shoes can be buttoned, garters fastened, and clothes put on in a very few minutes, *if* you watch yourself closely, and do everything in the easiest, shortest way. Of course, you have to think about what you are doing if you wish to do it neatly and quickly; or at least you must think about it until your muscles get so used to moving in the right way that they will do it without being reminded.

I have seen some children who take an hour or more to get dressed, and then they look only half dressed, for many of their

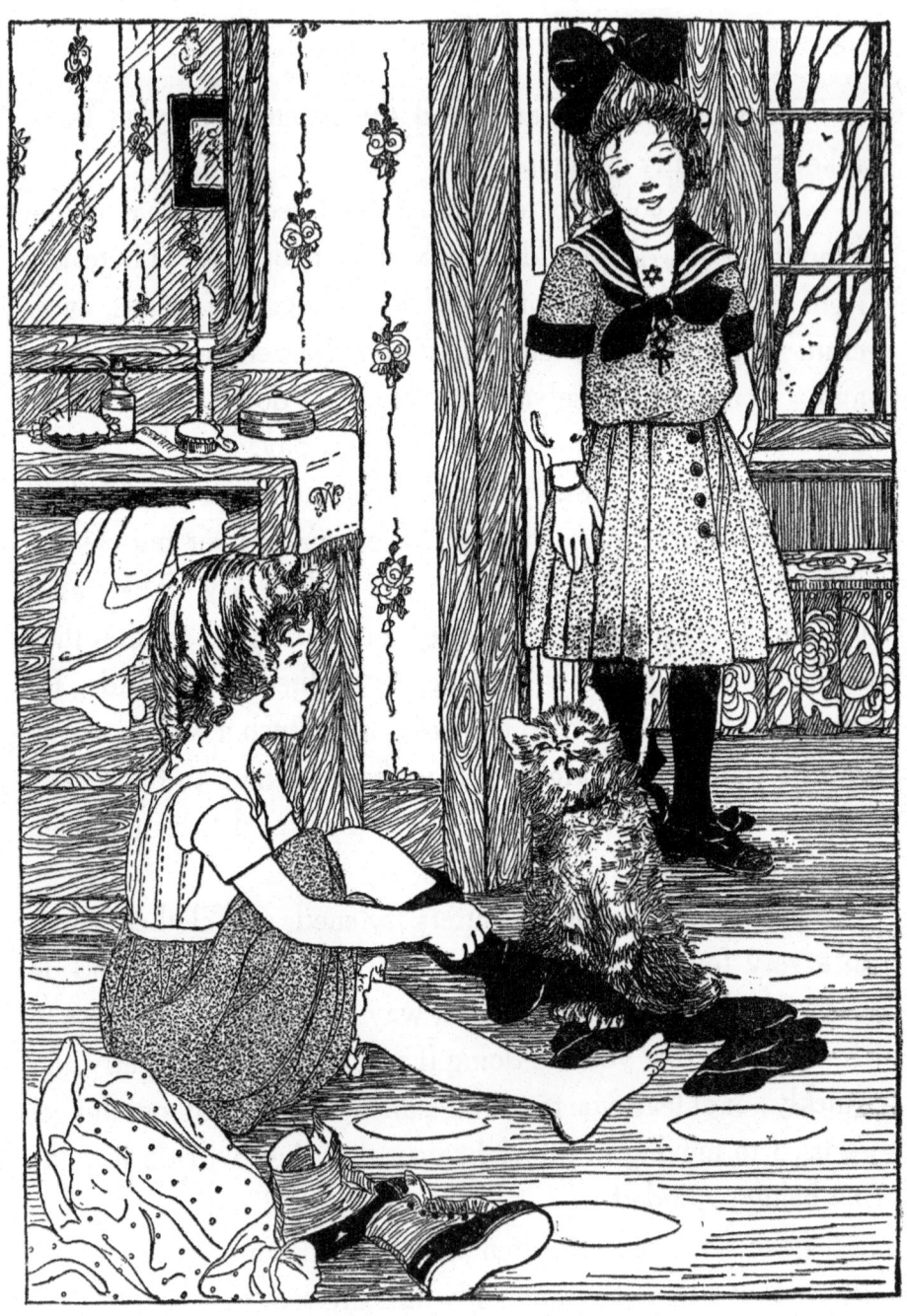

YOU CAN DRESS IN A VERY FEW MINUTES

things are put on crooked. But, I have seen others who make a game of getting dressed. They run races with their parents, with one another, or even with the clock. If you take off your clothes carefully at night, shake them well, turn them right side out, lay them down or hang them up where you can readily get at them in the morning, you can easily learn to put them on again in less than five minutes.

Many grown people whom I know, can do that part of their dressing in three minutes, in summer, and five in winter, and look as neat as if they came out of a bandbox. They have trained their muscles so well, that every motion is as exact and quick as that of a fine pitcher on a baseball team. The clothes go on just as they wish, and there are no wrong moves or hitches!

Many children whom I have seen consider it great fun to watch themselves every time they dress, to see how much better and quicker they can make their muscle servants obey them every day. It takes a great deal of practice before a child learns to dress very quickly, but as every child has to dress and undress at least three hundred and sixty-five times every year he lives, it will save him much time to learn to do it quickly and well right now.

About Doing Things

Let us suppose a child who likes to dawdle, look out of the window, play a little, grumble a little, who spends several minutes hunting around for missing shoes or stockings, buttons her clothes up crooked, and so has to unbutton and button them up again.

Such a child takes from half an hour to an hour, merely to put on her clothes,—for we are not talking now of washing, hair-combing, tooth-brushing or nail-cleaning.

In a year, a child who takes half an hour to dress every day, has spent one hundred and eighty-two and a half hours putting on her clothes. But the child who uses muscles and brains in such a way as to do the same work in ten minutes (it can be done in five), spends only a little more than sixty hours dressing.

The quick child, therefore, has about one hundred and twenty-two hours more to spend in play, or sleep, or anything he or she chooses to do, than the little slow poke! Now, it is just the same with everything else you undertake, and if you "use your brains," you can train your muscles to do the same work just a little quicker and better every day you live.

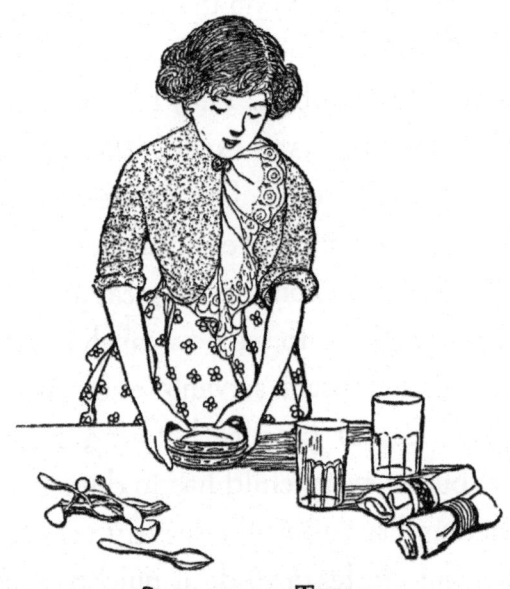

SETTING THE TABLE

Servants who set the table and wash the dishes three times a day, could save themselves ever so many steps, and gain much

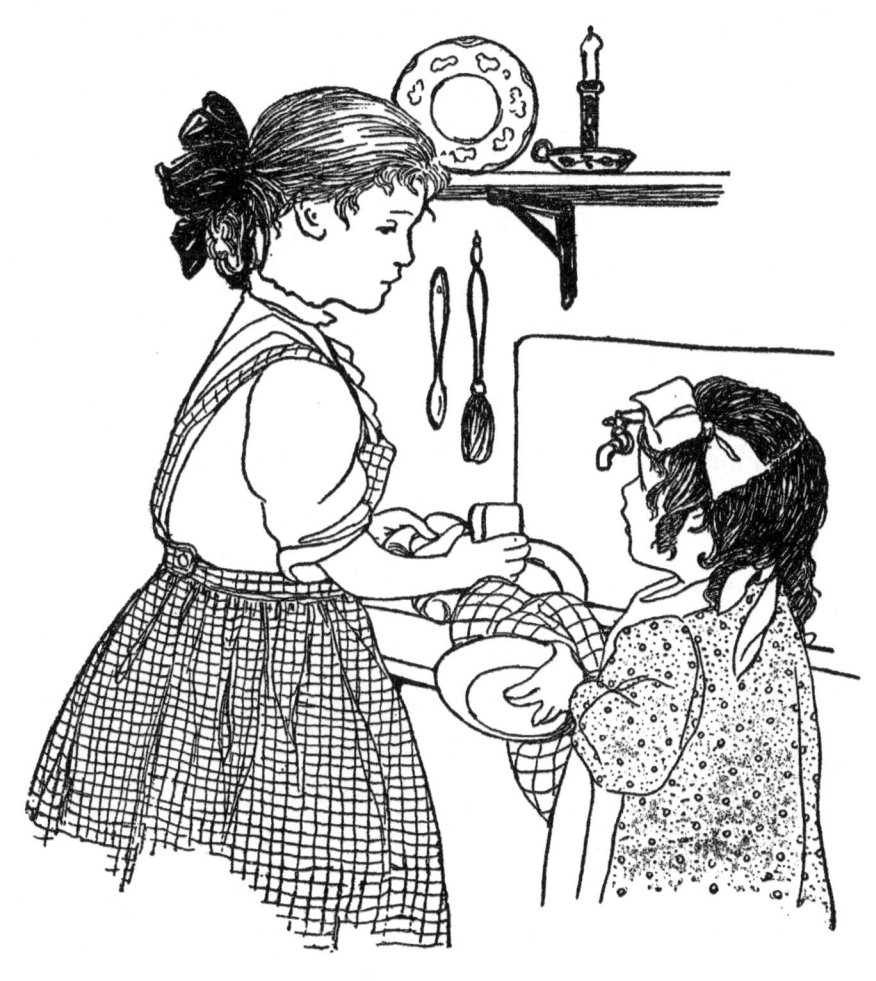

WASHING DISHES

time, if they only used their brains to train their muscles properly. But, a good part of the time they do not think of what they are doing, or only half think about it, and so their muscles work just as they please.

When the mistress has to do her servant's work, she is often surprised to see how quickly it can be done if she only thinks ahead, fixes things so as to have them handy, and takes as few steps, and makes as few unnecessary motions as possible.

If you have to set tables, wash dishes, dust rooms, empty ashes, cut wood, harness horses, run errands, or merely get ready for school, just watch yourself, and see whether you do it in the quickest, shortest, easiest and neatest way. I am sure most of you will find that you can teach your muscle servants new and better ways, which will be a great help later on.

I know a lady who has trained herself to do all her housework so beautifully and so quickly, that it seems almost like magic. She can go in the kitchen, cook the dinner, wash up all the dishes, pots and pans, and never get a speck of dust or the least little stain upon her best dress. She, her kitchen, and her whole house are always "as neat as wax."

This lady often says, laughing, that God gave her brains so that she could train her muscles. She also declares that she is far too lazy to be willing to spend all her time clearing up the mess she makes, and doing her daily housework. She is so smart and so quick, that she has plenty of time to sew, to go out calling, to play on the piano, to read and to paint, and still she really does much more work than many women I know, who spend all their time fussing over it.

Don't you think, therefore, that it pays to use one's brains to train one's muscles? If you use yours wisely while you are young, you can get your muscles in such good order by the time you are grown up, that you can do much in a short time with little fuss, or worry or fatigue.

A Baby's Training

Every baby moves his legs and arms about, clutches at all he sees, and pokes things into his mouth. That is baby's way of learning all about himself and about the strange things all around him.

Everything is new, and he has to find out for himself all about the world he lives in. A baby can learn all his first lessons far better than any one else can teach him. But when he gets old enough to notice what you are doing, and to imitate you, you can begin to teach him useful things just as easily as pretty tricks.

There was a baby once, who always wanted to go from one room into the other because the door between stood open the greater part of the time. This baby could creep very nicely, but as there was a high step between the two rooms, the other members of the family were kept running from morning till night to save her from a bad fall.

An older brother, who had to watch the baby,—and who did not enjoy being disturbed so often in his play,—finally used his brains to some purpose. He knew the baby liked to do whatever he did. So he set her down near the step, crawled towards it on his hands and knees, turned around, lay down flat on his stomach, and reached down first with one foot and then with the other. When both his feet were in the lower room, he sat down and crept on. As soon as the baby crept to the step, he turned her around, made her lie flat, put her feet down in the lower room, made her sit down, and then let her creep on.

Baby was delighted with this new game, which was repeated several times; after that, whenever she drew near the step, the big brother, instead of lifting her down as before, made her get down by herself, and before night baby could do it all alone, and enjoyed it as much as if it were a fine joke.

A few days later, to save himself the trouble of lifting baby *up* the step, this same brother showed her how to hold on by the door jamb, to raise one knee up on the step, then lie flat upon it, pull up the other foot, and creep on.

I also know a wise mother, who, instead of always giving her baby a spoon and a tin pan to play with, sometimes gave her a *loop* button hook. Several times she showed the baby how to hold this button hook, how to put it in the button-holes in her shoes, how to push it through them and over the buttons, and how to draw it back with one hand, while using the other to hold the button-hole in place.

Before long, this baby loved to play with the button hook and with her shoes, and, before she could walk, she had al-

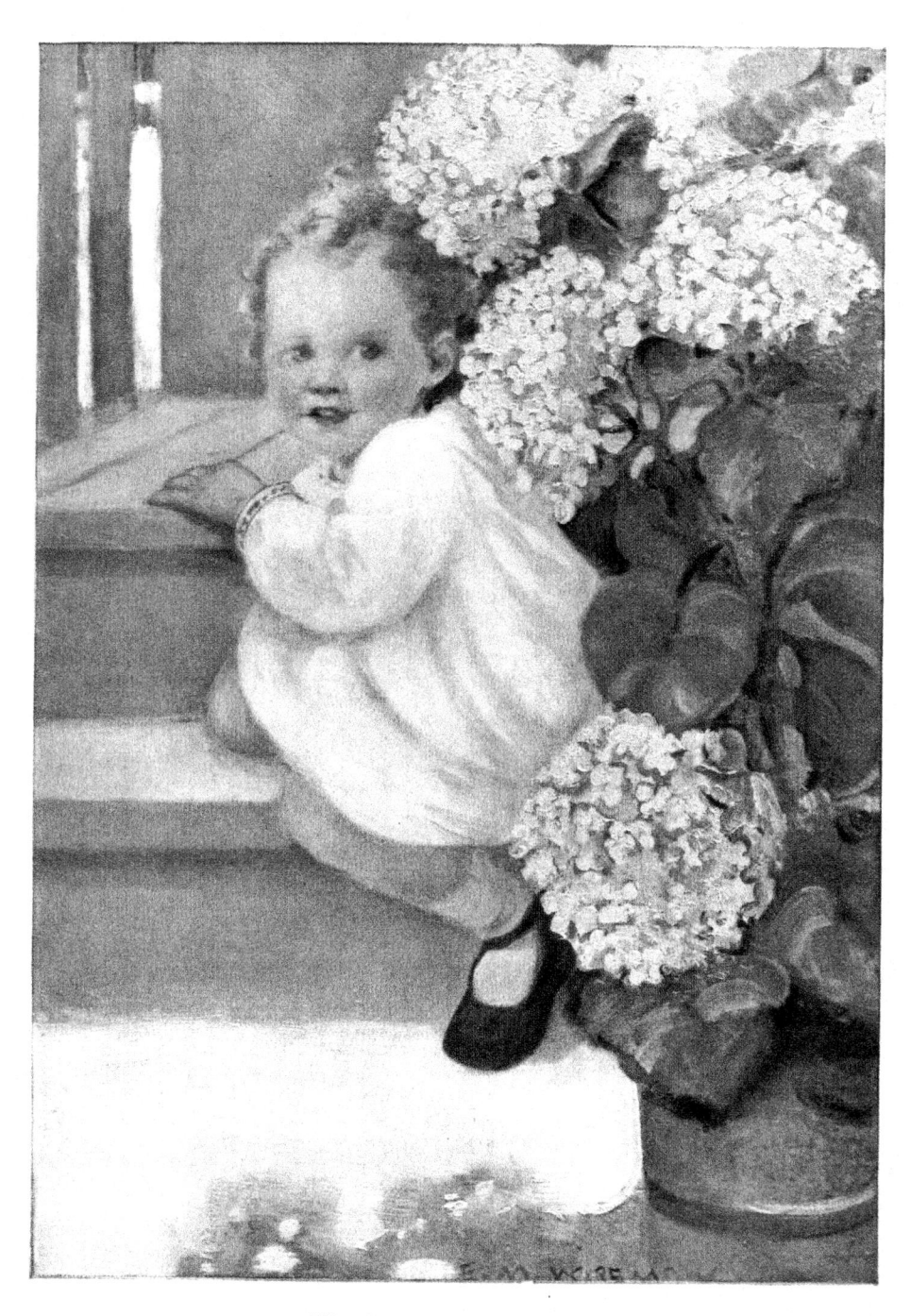

The Lesson of the Step

The Advantage of Well Trained Muscles

ready learned to button her own boots and loved to do it. In fact, it seemed such fine fun to her, that she gurgled and cooed while doing it, and laughed and shouted with glee as soon as it was all done.

It was such a nice game for baby, that her mamma had to unbutton her shoes time and again every day, so that she could button them up again. But the good mother knew that all this was fine practice for her baby's little muscles and so she did it gladly.

Later on, this mother was very happy indeed that her little girl could button her own shoes, at an age when most little ones two and three years older always had to have it done for them.

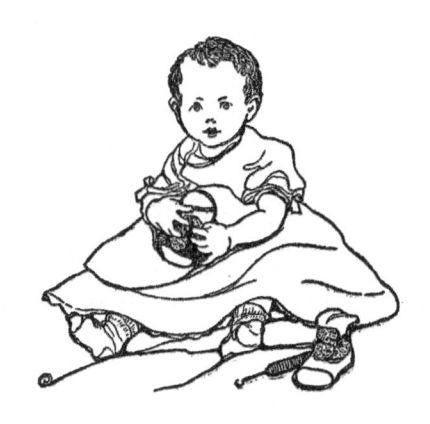

THE BABY WITH THE SHOE

It is very much kinder to show a little child carefully and patiently how to do a thing, and let him do it himself, than to do it for him. Of course, older people can do the thing much quicker and better, but baby's muscles have to be trained early and often if they are to make good servants for him later on.

THE ADVANTAGE OF WELL TRAINED MUSCLES

Children of your age can train the baby and themselves in many ways, and thus help their parents and teachers. They will then grow up clever and graceful, as well as strong and healthy men and women.

A boy or girl who learns to do any motion as quickly and well as it can be done, has gained just so much, and will be able to learn anything else much more easily. That is why every child should do school gymnastics and drill with all his heart, for all those motions are part of the training of his muscle servants.

In time of war or danger, men with well trained minds and muscles can quickly learn to do anything that is needful. But men who think little, and whose muscles are stiff and untrained, need a great deal of drilling before they are of any use.

For instance, a drill sergeant once had to teach some very stupid country boys how to march. He called "Right foot, left foot! Right foot, left foot!" until he was hoarse. But as these lads did not seem to know which foot was right and which was left, it was all in vain.

In despair, the sergeant finally bade these stupid youths tie a wisp of hay around one foot and a wisp of straw around the other.

Then he began the drill all over again saying: "Hay foot, straw foot! Hay foot, straw foot!" until he had taught them how to march properly. You see, these lads knew the difference between hay and straw, which they had often seen, and the sergeant had brains enough to find out this way to teach them what they had to learn.

The Advantage of Well Trained Muscles

In many schools, especially in cities, the children go through the fire drill very often, because the teachers know that when their muscles are thoroughly trained, they won't be likely to make any mistakes, and that all can get out of the building safely, even if it does catch fire.

Every child should therefore do his best to learn the drill well, and to obey every order as quickly and exactly as he can. Then, if the master of his little house keeps cool in time of danger, and does not bother the muscle servants by giving them wrong orders, all will be well, for the muscles know their duty and will be sure to do it.

The mother of a four year old boy trained her little son to drop anything and everything and run to her whenever she called him in a certain way. One day, she was out walking with the little fellow, who was standing some distance ahead of her.

They were near a field where some big boys were playing baseball. The mother saw a swift ball coming, and called her little son, who turned instantly and ran back to her. A second after he turned, the ball came whizzing across the walk, just at the spot where the child had been a moment before.

The mother said that nothing but his prompt obedience saved his life, for the ball would certainly have struck his temple with such force that the blow would have proved fatal. You can imagine how thankful that mother was to have trained her boy to obey right away. If she had allowed him to get in the habit of saying: "Yes, mamma, in a minute!" or of asking "Why?" before he obeyed, his life would have been lost.

When to Fight

While girls should train themselves, as soon as they can, to do all sorts of housework, boys can learn to drive in nails, and do all kinds of carpenter work deftly. Every kind of knowledge is useful some time or other, and I never heard any one regret that he knew how to do anything really well.

Many boys think only of growing very strong so as to lift great weights to surprise people, or to do other feats of strength. But such muscle training is not of much use, and the efforts made are likely to do great harm in the end. It is far, far better to be a skilful workman, in any trade, than a champion prize-fighter or a lifter of great weights.

If you have a chance to do so, boys, it is well to learn to fence

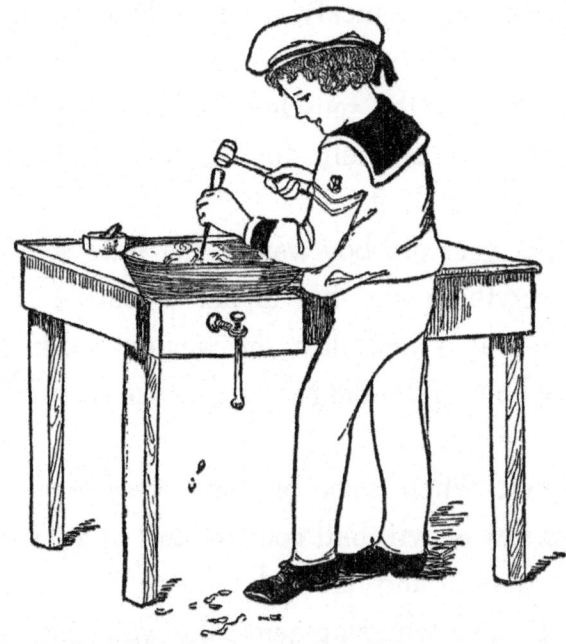

CARPENTER WORK FOR BOYS

and box. To fence or box well you have to give your muscles considerable training, which will make them strong and supple without straining them in any way.

Such training will besides enable a boy to hold his own, should he ever have to do any fighting. For there are times, you know, when even the most peaceable men or boys are forced to fight. I would advise any boy to keep out of a fight just as long as he can, but if he sees a big boy bully a little one, and cannot make him stop in any other way, he should give that bully a good thrashing.

In fact a man's or boy's strength is given him to defend himself against any attack, to fight for his country, and to protect girls, women, children, and all those who are weaker than himself.

The other day, I saw in a newspaper that a young woman was kept at work over hours and started to go home alone at ten o'clock at night. It was in a big city, and while she was waiting at the corner of the street for a car, a man stepped up and spoke to her.

This man must have been either drunk or bad, and he must have said something very horrid, for the young woman started back and looked around in a frightened way for a policeman. There was no officer in sight, and the rough man was just going to seize her arm, when another man, passing by, pounced upon the ruffian and gave him the thrashing he so richly deserved.

The newspaper said that the nice man was young and slender, and not nearly so tall and strong as the one he had attacked. But his muscles were well trained, and his indignation gave him the necessary strength to defend that woman.

He did not annoy her by speaking to her, or try to gain her notice in any way, but he held the ruffian down until she had stepped into her car and was out of harm's way. As there was no policeman there, at the time, to protect this lone woman, the young stranger did quite right to interfere and take the law into his own hands, and everybody admires him for it.

Every boy and man should learn to treat every girl and woman just as he would like other men and boys to treat his mother, his sister, or his wife. He should always be ready to protect them from rough men, and to give them any help in his power whenever they need it.

The boy heroes whom we hear about, who have saved people from drowning, from burning buildings, or who have snatched children or old people from in front of locomotives, or runaway horses, did not become heroes in a minute or even in a day.

When the moment of danger came, their minds and muscles, always on the lookout to help others, or to do a kind deed, merely acted in the usual way, without needing any prompting. But selfish and lazy boys never become heroes, for they are used to think of themselves only, and not of others, and their muscle servants have gotten into such bad habits, that they are quite useless in time of sudden need.

When to Fight

So, if you ever hope to be a hero, and to risk your own life without any hesitation to save another, you should begin right away to train yourself to think of others before you think of yourself. You should, besides, teach your muscle servants to be always ready and willing to serve others, and by and by they will be so used to doing it, that they will move in the right way almost before you know it.

QUESTIONS.—What covers all the framework of your house? What are muscles? What do the muscles bind together and move? How are orders carried from the master to the muscles? What are good ways in which boys and girls can develop their muscles? Do muscles have to be fed, and repaired? If so, how is it done? Should you give your muscles rest as well as exercise? Why is outdoor exercise better than any other? Can you train your muscles to be quick and precise, and can you explain how "practice makes perfect"? Are there right and wrong ways of doing everything, dressing, setting tables, etc.? What should you do with your clothes when you undress? Does it save time and trouble to train your muscle servants well? Should babies be patiently taught to do things for themselves? Of what advantage is it to go through gymnastic exercises and the fire-drill with all your heart, and to learn to do housework and carpentering, as well as to fence, box, and play tennis and ball?

CHAPTER IX

The Outside of Your House

WE have already talked a little about the skin, which covers all the outside, and lines all the inside of your little house. We have also noticed that the skin inside is not nearly so thick as the skin outside, and that you can plainly see the blood and flesh through it.

You know how delicate the inner skin is, and how careful we should be not to hurt it in any way. You are also aware of the fact that it is always kept moist and soft, and that it is fed and kept in good condition by the blood-boats, which supply it with all the food, air, and repairing materials it needs.

Now we are going to talk a little about the skin which covers the outside of your little houses. This is very much thicker than the inner skin, and seems quite different in make and in color. If you look at the skin on the back of your hand, you will notice a number of little marks upon it which look something like pin pricks.

These little marks, or holes in the skin, are called pores. Besides the big pores, which you can thus see in different parts of your body, there are ever and ever so many tiny little ones, which you cannot see unless you take a magnifying glass.

The Outside of Your House

The pores are the mouths or openings of many, many little tubes which run right down into your skin. Night and day, out of some of these tubes flows a fine oil (far too fine to be seen), which keeps the skin soft and smooth. We know that oil comes out of these pores, not only because some doctors have seen it with their microscopes, but also because our skin *feels* and often *looks* oily. It is often so oily that if you pour clear water upon it, the water will roll off without really wetting it. When we want to wet our skin therefore, we must first rub the oil off by means of soap and hot water.

There are millions and millions of pores in each human body, and while some pour out oil on the skin to keep it soft and smooth, others pour out water and refuse. The water which comes out of the pores generally comes in such very small drops that you cannot see it. It is like steam, and flies off in the air or is soaked up by our clothes.

But sometimes the pores send out so much water that it cannot all fly away and forms drops on the skin. Then we say that person is sweating or perspiring. The water which thus comes out on the skin helps to cool the body when it is too hot, so a person who perspires, suffers far less from *great* heat than one whose skin stays dry.

The body gets rid of much of its refuse by means of the skin. All the waste that is not cast out by the Garbage Can and Bladder Dwarfs, or blown out by the lung bellows, is sent out through the pores of our skin.

Each little pore, therefore, has its own share of work to do, and as long as it stays open it can work well. In fact the pores work night and day. They work when the master is asleep, just as well as when he is awake, and when they are all in good order they cast out nearly as much bad air, waste water, and other refuse, as is sent out of the body by other means, although you cannot see it.

How to Keep the Pores Open

You have all seen mucilage bottles, have you not? Did you ever notice that little by little as the sticky mucilage dried around the neck of the bottle, the opening got smaller and smaller? Indeed some mucilage bottles get all stopped up by the mucilage which dries and forms a kind of stopper in the neck of the bottle. When this happens, you can tip the bottle way over but no mucilage will come out.

Well, our pores are something like mucilage bottles. The water and refuse poured out of them dries around their edges, although you cannot see it without a magnifying glass. If this dry refuse is not washed away, so that the top of the tube (or the neck of the skin mucilage bottle) is kept quite clean and clear, the opening soon gets so stopped up that no oil, no water and no refuse can come out of it any more.

When this happens it is very bad indeed for the skin, and for the owner of the house. The little tubes go on bringing refuse and water to the top of the skin, which they wish to pour out, but they find the opening closed so tightly that they cannot do so.

This makes them very cross, for they all like to do their work as faithfully as they can. Then they try to make the master of the house understand that something is wrong, by sending him telegrams which make him feel a little uncomfortable. If this won't do, and the pore openings are not freed, the dirty skin often gets red and sore, or it gets rough and scaly, and the nerve telegrams keep telling the master that all is not right with the skin. The refuse, which cannot pass out through the skin when the openings are stopped up, is then carried back into the body, where the lungs and the kidneys have to take care of it, besides looking after their own share of waste.

As the body servants are all remarkably obliging and ready to help one another in time of need, the lungs and kidneys when thus called upon to take care of the skin refuse too, are very apt to say: "Poor skin, it must be sick, or it would surely do its own work. We must help it until it gets better."

Then the kidneys and lungs work harder still to do their own work and that of the skin as well. But if the skin does not soon get to work again, the lungs and kidneys get over-tired, and by and by they get very cross and begin to growl.

"Why does not that lazy skin get to work? We cannot go on forever doing its work as well as our own! Really, Master ought to see to this matter. It is not fair to overwork us in this way. We'll soon be sick too, if this goes on!"

A just master, who knows that his skin, lungs, bowels and kidneys each have their own work to do, and that if they do not do it nicely his house cannot be well kept, always tries to keep all these ways of removing waste in good order.

As you know, the kidneys are all right when the master eats plain, wholesome food, drinks plenty of pure water, does not catch cold and keeps cheerful and pleasant.

The lungs are all right as long as the master breathes plenty of nice fresh air, which has been sifted and warmed, and when he gives them plenty of room to swell out as much as they please, and sees that they are kept comfortably warm.

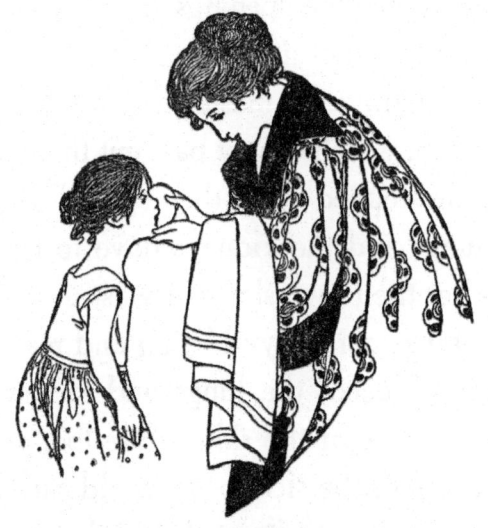

KEEPING THE SKIN HEALTHY

To keep the skin healthy, the master of the house must not only eat wholesome food, drink pure water, and breathe fresh air, but he must also keep every inch of it perfectly clean so that all the little pore openings will not be stopped up.

ABOUT BATHING

To keep your skin perfectly clean, and always in good con-

About Bathing

dition, you ought to take a good bath, or hard scrubbing, with hot water and soap at least once a week, washing every bit of your body thoroughly. If you perspire a great deal or if you do dirty work, it is often a good plan to put a teaspoonful of household ammonia to a basin of water before you begin to wash. Most people know enough to wash their faces and hands every morning; but this is not enough to keep our skin in good health. Faces and hands should be washed as often as needful to keep them nice and clean at all times. But, besides that, everyone should brush his or her teeth night and morning, wash the private parts carefully with soap and water, and take a sponge bath once a day.

Some people say they do not have time to do all this. Others declare that it would make them ill. Now, all these excuses are sheer nonsense, and only show that those who make them do not know how to wash quickly and well. Of course, if it takes them an hour every time they take a bath, I can readily understand that they cannot find the time. I can also understand that it makes them ill, for too much soaking is very bad for the body, while mere washing is good for it.

If you have a bathroom, with a tub and plenty of hot and cold water, you can soon learn to take a full bath, scrubbing every inch of your person with soap, rinsing yourself off carefully, and rubbing yourself dry, in about ten minutes. By taking fifteen minutes, you can empty and wash out the tub, so that the next person who wants to use it may find it nice and clean. In fact, you should always leave a bathroom as neat as you found it, and you can learn to do this so quickly and easily, that it will take very little time and be very little trouble.

If you have no bathroom, you can get just as clean, only perhaps not quite so easily or quickly, by washing your body piecemeal. Of course, for a thorough bath you need soap, hot water, and plenty of "elbow grease" as a good hearty scrubbing is called.

If you have done no dirty work at all, and only wish to get rid of the waste which you cannot see, but which has been cast out by your pores, a hard rub with a wet cloth, or sponging your body all over, will be enough every day, provided you take a good soap and hot water wash once or twice a week.

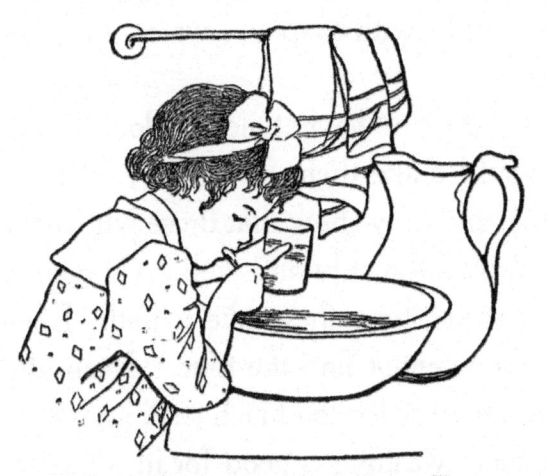

FIVE MINUTES DEVOTED TO YOUR TEETH

If you can strip entirely, and wring a rough bathing towel out in cold or warm water, you can soon find out the best way to hold it and to go to work so as to rub it hard all over your body in less than a minute. Then, with another towel, you can dry yourself and get into a fine glow in another minute, thus taking only two minutes for your whole bath.

Another five minutes devoted to your teeth, finger nails, and other parts of your body requiring special attention, will enable you to do all your washing in about seven minutes, and if you have short or only moderately long hair to brush and comb, you can get that in good order in five minutes or less.

Now, seven minutes for washing, five for your hair, and five to don your clothes, will enable you to get all ready in seventeen minutes, provided you waste no time, and train your muscle servants in such a way that they will always do their work both quickly and well.

Every one by rising early enough can surely afford to spend seventeen minutes for a thorough morning toilet. In fact they will be much better off if they do, than by taking five or ten minutes merely to get dressed, and washing only their faces and hands, as so many children and even grown people do.

But a person who begins the day in that way is beginning it all wrong. The skin, as you can easily notice, feels very different when dirty than when freshly washed. When clean, the pores are all open so the waste can be poured out freely, and the kidneys and lungs are not made to do extra work.

Washing Babies

If you keep your skin nice and clean by daily washing, it won't matter a bit if you do play in the mud and get very dirty.

That kind of dirt never hurts the body, nor stops up the pores, provided it does not stay on too long. The kind of dirt which does harm, is the waste from the body, which ought to be removed from the body every day if you wish to keep well.

Some old-fashioned folks fancy that washing is very bad for people, especially if they are young or sickly; but all the doctors will tell you that washing, on the contrary, helps every one to grow bigger and stronger. Of course, I do not mean *soaking* when I say *washing*. Soaking is good only for dirty clothes or for certain kinds of diseases, and children who stay in the water too long are sure to be ill.

Sick people need baths just as much or even more than well people. They should be washed very often if you wish them to get well. Although they cannot get into a tub, or take a sponge bath themselves, you can give them a thorough cleaning by wetting a small part of their bodies at a time, drying that spot nicely, and keeping all the rest carefully covered up in the meantime.

Babies, whose skin is so tender, ought to have a bath every day. If you are careful not to hurt or frighten them, and if both room and water are warm enough, the baby will be sure to enjoy his bath very much indeed.

All babies should be very carefully dried with a soft towel, looking out for all the little creases, and then gently rubbed, especially over the chest and back. If baby's skin looks red and sore in the creases, you should dust it over with a little pure corn-starch, or baby powder, or put some vaseline upon it. But

Washing Babies

if you are careful to keep your baby dry, to wash and dry him every time you change his diapers, and to use clean diapers only, it is not likely that any powder will be needed to keep his skin healthy.

If baby's skin is not kept in first-class condition by frequent baths, his tiny pores (you cannot see them) will all be stopped up. His kidneys and lungs will thus have more than their share of work to do, and they will soon get tired. Neither skin, nor kidneys, nor lungs, can be in good health and temper unless each of them gets just the right treatment, and to treat your skin rightly you must keep it clean.

I know some children, who, when sent to wash their hands, always wash the insides or palms only, and forget the backs of their hands and fingers. A good way to go to work is to put water in a basin and rub some soap on the palms of both hands. Then put down your soap. Clasp one hand tightly around each finger of the other hand in turn, and rub that finger hard backward and forward.

When you have gotten all the fingers and the thumb of that hand clean in this way, rub the back of that same hand. Then clasp your wrist and screw that back and forth in your hand a few times. A good rub to the arm up to the elbow, will make that arm and hand quite clean.

Next, soap the clean hand, and give the one you first used as a rubber a good hard scrubbing in the same way. Then take your nail or scrubbing-brush, wet it, rub soap on it, and scrub your finger nails very hard, holding fingers and thumbs close together against the bristles.

A good rinsing and drying after this operation—which you can learn to do very quickly with practice—will leave you with nice, clean hands. Then, if you take a wooden toothpick or an orange stick, and use it to remove any dirt which may be left, from under your finger nails, you will be ready to go to school, or to sit down to table with really clean hands.

About Lunches

Every man, woman and child should always be careful not to eat or touch any kind of food unless his or her hands are perfectly clean. In the dirt and dust which we get on our hands, there are many little seeds of disease. If we swallow these, they may find a little corner in our bodies where they can grow, and they will soon spread from there and make the whole body very sick.

The other day I was watching a house painter. He had been at work, and his hands were dirty and all daubed over with paint. When the noon whistle blew, he dropped his brush and took his dinner pail. As there was no water to be had, I wondered how he was going to manage to eat his dinner without its tasting of paint and dirt.

So I watched him open his pail and take out a parcel all wrapped up in a nice white napkin. He carefully undid this napkin, and folded it around his sandwiches, which he handled in such a neat, deft way that his dirty fingers never once touched his food or came near his mouth except when all covered by the nice clean napkin.

You see, that man knew that paint and dirt mixed with his food, would make him ill, and besides, although he had to work at a dirty trade, he was a nice clean fellow. As he could not wash before dinner, he did the next best thing. Still, I am quite sure that man had a good scrubbing when he got home before he sat down to the family supper table.

Some of the men who do the dirtiest work are really very clean, far cleaner than any of those who look much neater, but who do not take as good care of their bodies, or keep their skin in fine condition by plenty of washing.

Many of the school children can learn a useful lesson from this house painter, as far as their own lunches are concerned. Some mothers have time to prepare the children's lunch nicely, but many boys and girls have to get their own ready or go without any. If you cannot have nice clean napkins or oiled paper, you can save up all the clean tissue and brown paper which comes into the house for future use.

Cut this paper into squares of the right size, and wrap up each article of food separately, so that when you open it in school, it will tempt you to eat heartily and will not disgust others. Some of the teachers who are on duty during the noon hour have told me that they were often unable to touch their own lunches, because they had been so sickened by the sight of the messes which some of the children had.

Why not cut up your meat into small pieces, or mince it fine before you put it between slices of buttered bread? Then, wrap your meat sandwiches in a separate piece of paper from your jam sandwiches. Cover your custard cup neatly with a

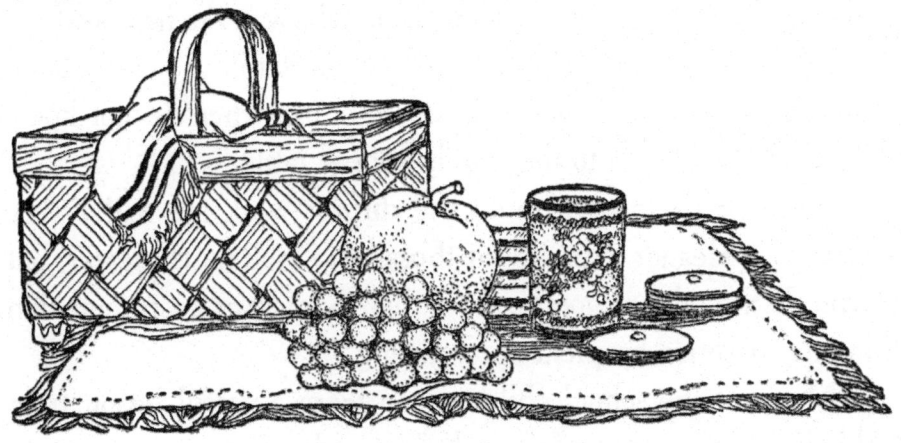

A NICE SCHOOL LUNCHEON

paper; wash your fruit clean and dry it nicely before you wrap it up too. Then pack your lunch in a tidy way in a box or basket, so that it will be as nice when you open it as when it was put in.

Of course, in every school there are washstands where you can wash your hands before and after meals. If you are neat you will do so, and use a towel of your own which you keep in your desk for that purpose. Every person should have his or her own private towel, and use no other, whether at home, at school, in the office or shop. It is the only safe rule to follow, if you wish to run no risks of catching some nasty skin or eye disease, and, as you know, one cannot learn good habits too early.

No Right to be Dirty

In all my life I never heard of but one person who injured her health by too much washing. But I have heard of and seen any number of people who neglected their skin, and let it get in a shameful condition, which—although they did not know it or would not believe it if told—was one of the main reasons why they so often felt poorly.

Dirty people not only harm themselves, but they are very offensive to clean people. One dirty man or woman in a street car, in a stage, or on a train, can poison all the air, and make all the other passengers very uncomfortable. So you see, even if we do not respect our own bodies, and wish to keep them clean for our own sakes, we ought to be clean for the sake of others.

This is a free country, and every one has a right to live and act as he pleases, *provided* he does not interfere with the rights of other people. But, no one has the right to poison the air others breathe, so you see no one has really the right to be anything but clean if he wishes to live near other people.

In cities, the board of health arrests people whose *houses* are not kept clean, for we now know that dirt breeds disease. Before long, there may even be laws which will make it right to arrest dirty persons, and all those who smell bad.

Meantime, each child who reads this book can see to it that his own skin is daily washed and thus kept in such good order, that never mind what work he may do, or how dirty he may get during the day, he will never be really offensive to any one, and can always respect himself.

Because our body is always casting out refuse night and day, through the pores, the clothes we wear next the skin should be changed and washed very often. It is always best to have woolen, or cotton and woolen underclothes, and of rather loose than tight texture and fit. You should take off these garments every night, give them a good shaking, so that the dry waste can fly off, and hang them up to air during the night.

Then you should put on clean night clothes, which you can take off in the morning, shake in their turn, and hang out of the window to air thoroughly before you put them away for the day.

Underclothes and night clothes should be changed and washed at least once a week. The bed sheets, too, should be well shaken and aired every day, and changed and washed quite frequently. Much of our skin waste can be found on our sheets, as you can see for yourself if you shake your sheet against the light or in a sunbeam. A white cloud of dust will fly off from it. This dust is body or skin refuse, and like all waste it should be gotten rid of, and not kept near the body any longer than needful.

As every one likes to appear as well as possible, I need not say much about your outside clothes. But remember, it is far

No Right to be Dirty

more important for your health that your underclothes should be clean, dry, well aired and changed often, than that the

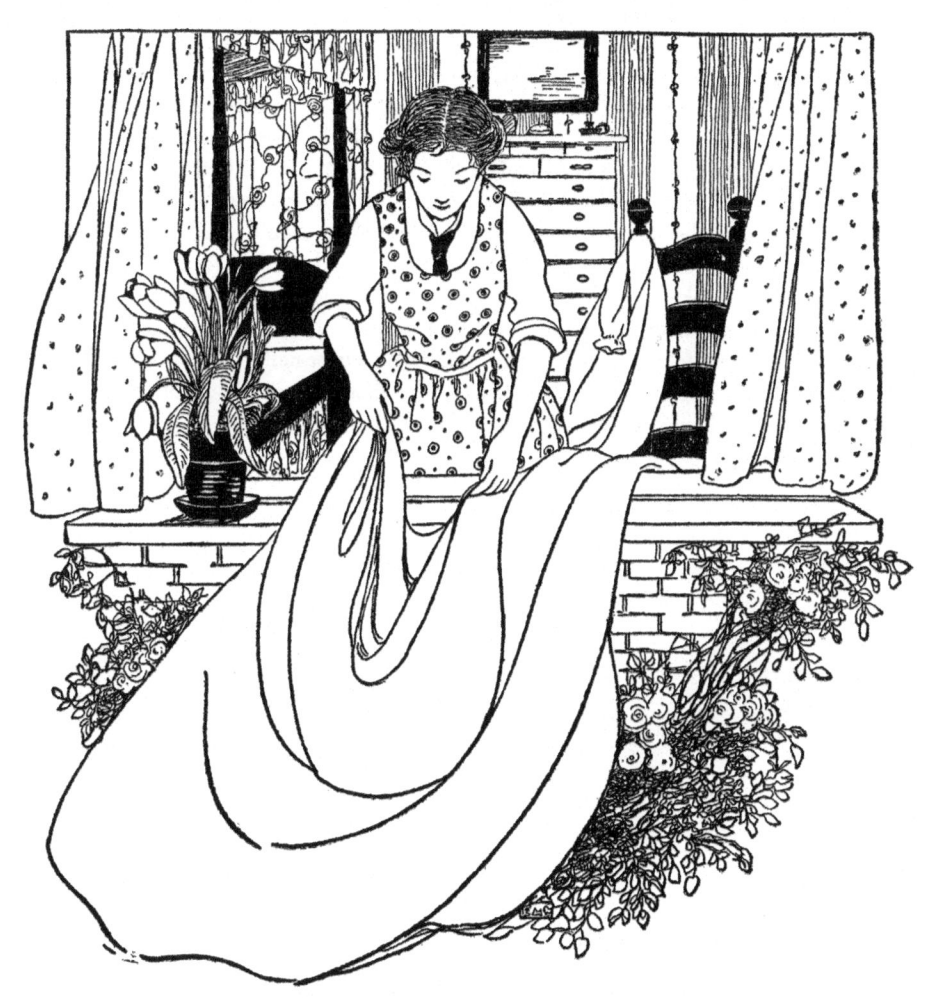

BED CLOTHES SHOULD BE AIRED DAILY

clothes which everybody can see shall be handsome. Now that clothes are cheap and easy to buy ready made, there is no excuse for any one to be dirty, and good underwear can be bought for a few cents.

QUESTIONS.—What covers all the outside and inside of your house? What is the difference between the outside and inside covering? What are the little holes in the skin called, and what do they do night and day? When the pores send out water enough to be seen, what do you call it? Is all the body waste thrown out of your house by the Garbage Can and Bladder Dwarfs? What is the difference between open and closed pores and which are best for you to have? What must the master do to keep the skin working nicely? How often should you wash the different parts of your house? If you have trained your muscles well and do it every day, how long does it take for a bath? Should you give more time to teeth, hands and hair? Should the baby be bathed and kept clean? Can you show me how you should go to work to have really clean hands and finger-nails? Why should your hands be clean before you touch food, and why should your school lunch be neatly packed? How should you care for your bed clothes, and are sun, air, and a shaking good for them?

CHAPTER X

BEING CAREFUL FOR THE SAKE OF OTHERS

IN olden times, when the father of the family had to grow all the cotton and flax, and to raise all the wool used for garments, when the mother had to clean it, spin it, weave it, dye it, and make it up into clothes, with no help of sewing or any other of our fine machines, it is no wonder that people had too few clothes to change as often as good health requires.

Even forty years ago, during our civil war, cotton was so very dear, that a handkerchief cost nearly a dollar. It is no wonder, therefore, that people who lived in those days could not, many of them, afford to buy handkerchiefs, and thus got into the habit of blowing their noses with their fingers.

Now that you can buy a handkerchief for two cents,—if need be,—there is no excuse whatever for not having one always on hand, and a clean one at that. All children should therefore learn very early to have a handkerchief, and to use it to keep their noses and mouths clean, and to wipe off their fingers when necessary.

A child who does not have a handkerchief, and use it freely instead of snuffing or sniffling, has not been well brought up, and should be taught good habits as soon as possible. All the children who read this book are, of course, old enough to know how to use their handkerchiefs, but they should also be careful to teach their little brothers and sisters how to use them too, so that they can keep clean, and never present the disgusting sight of a dirty nose. Little children can be nicely trained in this matter very early, provided their older brothers and sisters are careful and always give them a good example.

Boys may think it is manly to imitate some old workmen they have seen, and to blow their noses with their fingers. These boys evidently do not know that if handkerchiefs had been as cheap and plenty when those men were young, as they are now, these men would never have gotten into habits which shock people now because they are neither clean nor nice.

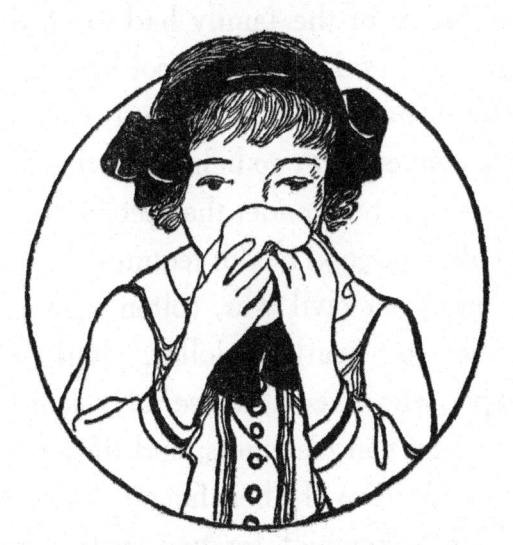

Use Your Handkerchief

A Wise Law

People should also always use their handkerchiefs whenever they have anything in their mouths which they wish to

A Wise Law

spit out. Doctors have found out, within the last few years, that spittle often contains many little disease seeds or germs. When the spittle dries, these little germs are set free, caught up by the wind, and begin to fly about.

Then they can be drawn right into other people's lungs, where they often find little corners where they can settle down comfortably and grow until they cannot be driven out any more. The person in whose lungs they thus settle, soon grows weak and ill, and thousands of people die every year from disease caught in just this way.

Because the spittle from one sick person—who may not know he is sick—can make many others ill, the laws in certain cities and states forbid spitting in the street, in any conveyance, or in a public building. Any one who disobeys this law is likely to be arrested or fined.

I am sure that all you children will now see how wise this law is, and how important it is for public health that no one should ever be allowed to break it. Our duty is, therefore, to watch over ourselves closely, to see that we always spit in our handkerchiefs only, to train all the younger children to do so too, and help the police in every way to enforce a law which was made to guard us one and all from a deadly enemy.

If there is a consumptive person in your house, he or she should not only sleep in a bed but in a room alone. Besides, there should always be plenty of fresh air in this room.

Even a person only a little consumptive should never spit into anything but a paper handkerchief, which should be used only a few times, and then burned, so as to make sure that all the little disease seeds are killed right away.

If cotton or linen handkerchiefs are used, they should always be boiled. After clothes have been thoroughly boiled they can always be used again by any one without danger. In that way only, one can make sure that all the little disease seeds are killed before they can do any one else any harm. If everybody were really careful about these things, there would not be nearly as many sick people in the world as there are now, and everybody would therefore be much happier.

Catching Diseases

There are many, many "catching" diseases, a few of which every one is likely to take some time in his life. Some are caught by breathing in little disease seeds, or by catching a sick person's breath, and some are taken by touching a sick person's skin or some article of dress he or she has worn. Chicken-pox, measles, whooping-cough, mumps, scarlet-fever, diphtheria and smallpox are all diseases which spread very rapidly, unless great care is taken to prevent their doing so.

While chicken-pox, measles, mumps and whooping-cough are quite common, and not all dangerous in themselves, children often die from these very diseases, if they do not receive proper care while they have them.

Catching Diseases

You may think your mamma very unkind to keep you in bed or in a dark room when you perhaps hardly feel sick at all. But mamma knows that if you catch cold while suffering from any of these diseases, you may be very ill indeed, so ill that may be you will die, or be sickly all the rest of your life.

Your mother also knows that a child who has the measles, should always be kept in a dark room, for if the light shines into your eyes while you are thus ill, you may have weak or sore eyes for many years afterwards.

Scarlet-fever, diphtheria, and smallpox are much worse diseases than measles or whooping-cough, and for that reason all the doctors and health boards watch over those who have them. They do so because they wish to prevent their being careless, or doing anything which would spread those diseases.

Every person in our country should feel it a sacred duty to be as careful as possible not to give any sickness to any one else. A child with the mumps, the whooping-cough or any other catching disease, should be taught to keep far away from all other children until all danger of giving it to them is entirely over.

It is because your teachers do not wish the other children to run any risk of getting sick, that they send you home whenever they think you may have any catching disease, or when they know there is such an illness in your house, and fear that you may bring it to others in your clothes.

There are also many catching skin and eye diseases; so if

you see a child with sore eyes, or a blotchy or pimply skin, you had better keep far away from him, until your mother can find out whether it is quite safe for you to sit or play together. The best way to avoid being ill, or catching unpleasant things, is to keep well and happy yourself, to be perfectly clean, not to take cold, and to stay far away from any one from whom you could catch anything unpleasant.

ABOUT WET FEET

People can get very sick if they are not careful to keep warm and dry when it is cold or rainy. If you have not clothes enough to keep warm, just fold some old newspapers around your back and chest, and wear them between layers of your clothes.

Paper is the warmest and lightest thing any one can wear, and for that reason many poor people make paper comfortables for their beds by sewing a number of newspapers together. Sometimes, to prevent these newspapers from tearing, they are fastened between two thicknesses of calico. In that way fine large comfortables can be made for less than twenty-five cents apiece.

When you get wet, or even damp, you should always change your clothes right away. If you cannot do so, keep moving briskly until you have a chance to change them, for you will be far less likely to take cold if you keep your body warm inside by plenty of exercise.

About Wet Feet

Your feet especially should always be dry, so do not grumble any more when mamma tells you to change your shoes and stockings. Instead of pouting, see how quickly you can obey, and find out in how short a time a smart boy or girl can get out of wet shoes and stockings and into dry ones. Some people can do it inside of two minutes; can you beat that record? Try it next time your feet are wet and find out.

In driving past a poor cottage one cold day a lady saw several little bare-footed children. She felt sorry for the poor little things when she saw their blue legs and feet, and bought them each two pairs of strong shoes and thick stockings. The

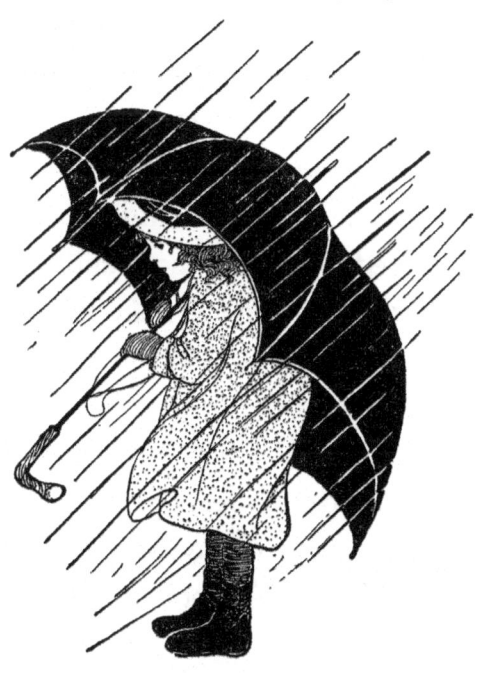

KEEP DRY IN WET WEATHER

children and their mother were delighted, and every time the lady passed the little ones waved their hands and pointed joyfully at their nicely clothed feet.

But one day no children were playing in front of the cottage door. The lady was so surprised that she got out of the carriage and knocked at the door When the mother opened, there was an awful scowl on her face and when the lady asked: "Where are the children, are they sick?"

"Sick! Sure and it's almost dead they are!" answered the woman angrily. "And it's all your fault! They never were sick before, and now they all have croup, and the doctor says it's all because they wore wet shoes and stockings!"

"Why didn't you make them change their shoes and stockings, if their feet were wet?" asked the lady. "I gave each child two pairs of shoes and stockings on purpose."

But the woman would not listen. She ran into the house, gathered up all the shoes and stockings and threw them at the lady's feet, saying, "Take back your old shoes and stockings, and don't come here any more trying to kill my children!" Then she slammed the door in her face. Do you think this woman was right? What do you think she should have done?

To keep one's feet dry, it is best to wear thick shoes, leggings, and rubbers in stormy weather. But these should be worn only out of doors. As soon as you get in the house, always be sure to take off your rubbers, or else your feet will grow tender and sore, and you will be far more likely to catch cold and be ill.

You see, as you are the owners and keepers of your little houses, you always have to bear in mind how you can best keep them in first-class order and repair, so that you won't need to be ashamed of their appearance or feel uncomfortable.

Any master who lives in a badly kept house, can neither be comfortable nor happy, and his house will soon go to pieces.

Besides he is not faithful, for God has given each of us a house to be used but not to be abused.

THE HAIR AND FINGER NAILS

The hair which grows so thickly all over your head has to be kept in good order, if you do not wish to look like a savage or a Shetland pony. Hair gets dirty as well as the skin, and needs a good washing every once in a while.

Boys who keep their hair short all their lives, have no trouble in washing it. They should give their heads a good scrubbing at least once a week, and oftener if they work at some dusty or dirty trade.

A good combing and hard brushing will keep your hair in order the rest of the time. It does not need to be plastered down with hair oil or water to look neat. In fact, it will be much better for your hair and scalp (the skin on your head), if you are satisfied to comb and brush and wash your hair, whenever it needs it, and to leave it alone the rest of the time.

Each hair is supplied with its own little oil-can, hidden under the skin, which pours out just enough of the right kind of oil to keep it in good condition, and you do not need to add any other kind of grease. The shorter a boy keeps his hair, the easier it will be to keep it clean. For that reason soldiers and officers always keep it cut as closely as possible.

Girls who have long hair ought always to cover it with a cap or handkerchief, while they are sweeping or dusting or doing any other dirty work. If they are careful about this matter, their hair will keep clean longer, and will not need to be washed so often.

A girl's hair needs washing only about once a month, provided she is very careful when sweeping, does not perspire much, and combs and brushes it thoroughly morning and evening.

When the hair is long, or curly and thick, it is apt to tangle pretty badly. The quickest and easiest way to get the snarls out, without breaking or pulling out any hair, is to hold the hair firmly in one hand, and the comb in the other.

Begin within an inch or two of the ends, and comb down. When the comb runs smoothly through that part of the hair, start an inch or two further up, and again comb downward. By proceeding thus, you take out the tangles little by little, and really get through your task much sooner and with far less discomfort.

Nicely combed, smoothly brushed and neatly braided or twisted hair always looks pretty. But flying locks are never tidy, and curls and frizzes, not of nature's own making, are a great waste of time and patience.

You should always do your hair up neatly before leaving your room in the morning, and if you want it to look nice and last long, you should brush and comb it also before you go to bed, and see that it is done up securely so as not to be in your way and not to get badly tangled while you are asleep.

The Hair and Finger Nails

Finger nails need brushing almost every time you wash your hands, and they need cleaning whenever they are the least bit dirty. Still, you should never clean them in public, but do this in your own room, in the toilet room, or when you are sure you are alone. Never mind what dirty work you have to do, you can, if you like, have clean hands and finger nails when your work is over.

Finger and toe nails should be kept just short enough to come even with the tops or ends of fingers and toes. It is always best to cut them with sharp scissors, and a little practice will soon enable you to cut those on your right hand as well as on your left.

When cutting your finger nails, you may, if you choose, round off the corners. You should carefully push back the skin at the bottom or root of the nail so the little half moon shows. If you push back the skin in this way you won't have any hang nails.

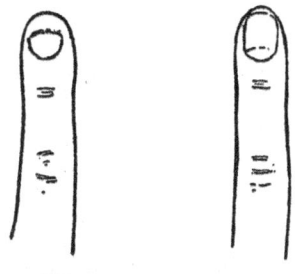

WHICH NAIL LOOKS LIKE YOURS?

As your shoes press on either side of your feet you should cut your toe nails straight across and *not* round off the corners. If you do, you may suffer from ingrowing toe nails which hurt very badly.

There are many children,—and some grown ups,—who, I am sorry to say, bite their finger nails. This is a very bad and unpleasant habit, which may harm them and which also makes other people very uncomfortable.

As our hands touch everything, they are, of course, most likely to get dirty and to pick up tiny disease seeds, which, if we put our fingers to our lips, may be swallowed and perhaps make us ill. Besides, finger nails are very rough, and the sharp parings may damage the tender skin of the stomach and pipes through which they have to pass before they can be cast out of the body as waste.

Next time you cut your nails just take a paring and jab yourself with it. You will soon find out that it is pretty sharp and that it can pierce even the tough skin on your hand. So, finger nails, if swallowed can punch tiny holes in your inner tubes and do lots of mischief down there. Doctors will even tell you of cases where children have died merely because they had the bad habit of biting their finger nails and swallowing the little bits in their mouths.

Now any bad habit *can* be broken if you try hard enough all the time, and surely any sensible boy or girl will understand that this habit is not only offensive to others, but very dangerous to the one who practices it, and will therefore try to get rid of it as soon as possible.

QUESTIONS.—What use do nice children make of a handkerchief? Why are people told not to spit in cars and on the street? How are catching diseases taken? In measles, mumps, chicken pox, or whooping cough, why should care be used so children won't catch cold and why are they in some cases kept in a partly dark room and not allowed to read? Is it wise to keep on wet or damp shoes and stock-

The Hair and Finger Nails

ings? Why should you always take off your rubbers in the house? How can you keep short hair and long hair in good order? How should a tidy boy's or girl's hair look? How should girls protect their hair from dust while sweeping? How can you keep finger and toe nails in order? Is it nice to clean your finger-nails in public? Is it right for children to bite their finger-nails? What do you suppose the Stomach Dwarf says when bits of finger-nail come down the staircase? What part of the body can these sharp bits damage?

CHAPTER XI

YOUR CENTRAL OFFICE AND ITS STORES

WE have already talked considerably about the master who dwells in each human house, be it little or big, pretty or homely, good or bad. This master is the real person, the mind, or spirit, which does all the thinking, planning and directing.

House masters are as different as the places they dwell in, but each one has to stay in the house where God placed him so long as life lasts.

Most of us believe that when the human house is worn out, and falls into decay, God allows the master to move out and occupy a better one, provided he has shown he is fit to be trusted by taking proper care of this one and making the best use of it.

As we have already said, each master lives in the top story of the house, where he can look out of the two windows, and see all that is going on. His whole house is very wonderful, but the most wonderful and interesting part of all, is surely that in the bone box called the skull.

The master's office is in there, so are the main telegraph and telephone stations of the house. From these stations start any number of telegraph wires—or nerves. Nerves are tiny white cords, so small that you cannot see them, except when many of them run along side by side, and thus form thick cables of many fine wires or threads.

Although many of these little telegraph wires start out and run to every part of the face, the greater part of them run down your back together, and then branch off from there to all the different parts of your body inside and out.

The biggest nerve cable, (which is made up of ever so many fine threads) runs right through the little bones which form the spine, stringing them all together like beads.

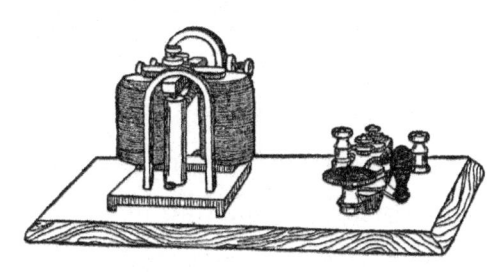

A TELEGRAPH INSTRUMENT

With bones all around it—bones which have many joints and can therefore bend almost any way you please—the nerves of the spine are so well protected, that they can do their work without running much risk of being broken or damaged.

You can see in pictures just how little branch telegraphs start off, here and there, along the main line. But pictures only show the biggest nerves or wires. If they tried to show you all the fine little ones, there would be such a network of white lines that you could no longer see where any of them went and would be greatly bewildered.

There are so many nerves, because every hair on our body, every pore in our skin, every little wee bit of tube, and every scrap of muscle or bone has its own nerve, so as to send a message if necessary. Night and day, as long as we live, messages flash back and forth along these little nerves. Not a breath is drawn, not a motion is made, not a heart beat takes place, without the nerves sending orders to have it done and reporting just how it was done.

If the poor master of the house had to direct every breath, every heart beat, and all the other wonderful things which are always going on night and day in his house, he would have no chance at all to sleep, to think, or to enjoy himself. So the greater part of the work in his house is done by clever servants, who do not trouble him in any way.

There is, for instance, a servant in the breathing telegraph office. He sends all the orders about breathing, year in and year out, and sees to it that all goes on well in his department, whether the master is watching him or not. Sometimes the master asks his servant how things are running, orders him to take extra long breaths, makes him keep the bellows very full of air, or empty them quickly or slowly. But generally the master lets the breathing servant manage his work just as he pleases.

As long as the master does not wear tight clothes (which prevent the ribs from rising, and the muscle wall from sinking when the bellows fill with air), and as long as he can get plenty of nice pure air, the breathing servant is quite happy, and need not consult his master. But when the air is too damp or too cold, when it is smoky or not pure, or when there is not room enough for the bellows to open wide and receive all the air they can hold, this servant gets sorely troubled. Then he sends messages to the master, who can pay heed to them or not just as he chooses. But if the master does not listen to them, he is not doing his duty, and soon all will go wrong in his little house.

There is another station, where a servant receives all the messages from the Pumping Dwarfs, and gives them the necessary orders. In another place all the messages from the stomach are received and answered. There is also one for the skin, one for the kidneys, one for the eyes, one for the ears, and so on, because each bone, each muscle, each cell, each tube, and all the different parts of the body we have mentioned, have nerves which run straight to certain stations.

As all these stations are managed by skilful servants, the house master does not need to bother about them at all. Besides, they are all connected with the main office, the brain, where he sits, and the minute anything is wrong, or needs his attention, he knows perfectly well that those trusty servants will send him notice.

About Nerves

If the master is clever, knows how his house is made, what his servants need, and how his machinery can be kept in the best order, he can easily find out what is wrong, whenever he receives a message saying that things are not running smoothly.

When any one knows just what is wrong, he generally

knows how to set it right, and how to prevent any further trouble of the same kind. A good master can, therefore, see not only that the damage is repaired as soon as possible, but that the same accident does not occur again.

But a stupid, careless, or ignorant master, gets quite bewildered, whenever any of his servants send word that anything is out of order. He does not try to find out what is the matter, or to set it straight, but only growls and grumbles because he is disturbed and made uncomfortable. When too unhappy or uneasy, he sends for a doctor to set things right for him, but often a little common sense, used in time, would have made everything right, and prevented all this fuss and damage.

The nerves, like the muscles, are apt to get very tired, for they too, use up a little of their material every time they do anything. Still, if the blood-boats bring them plenty of wholesome food, fresh air, and other materials for repair, they will keep well, work well, and be happy, provided you give them enough rest. In fact, people with really healthy nerves, are those who never know that they have any, that is to say who never *feel* them in any unpleasant way.

If the nerves do not get food, air, or rest enough, or if they are squeezed too tightly, or hurt in any other way, they are very likely to be unhappy and ache. When they feel very badly, they make the master of the house so uncomfortable, that he knows there is something wrong, and that he has nerves. Often, other people know it too, and then they call him nervous.

About Nerves

When a grown person, or a doctor, talks about nerves or nervousness, it is generally all right, but when children complain that they are nervous it is all wrong. Your fathers and mothers, who often have to be up all night with sick children, who have to work all day, look after the housekeeping, make and mend all your clothes, plan how to make a little money buy all you need, and do many other things, are of course very tired. They wear out every day more nerve material than food, air and the little rest they get, can repair. As you can plainly see, they cannot be anything but nerve-tired or nervous.

But children, who sleep all night, who have no cares, and who do very little hard work, have no excuse whatever for having tired nerves. When such children are nervous, you may be very sure it is either because they are not eating the right kind of food at the right time, because they play too hard, read too exciting stories, or perhaps because they do not get enough air or exercise.

A little girl who was fond of putting on airs, once told her mamma she was far too nervous to go to school, but quite well enough to go to a party! The mother, who knew that when children talk about nerves it is all nonsense, and only means that they are spoiled, answered: "You nervous! What nonsense. Don't you know that nerves don't grow until you are forty!"

Her little girl never talked about her nerves again. Now, that mother knew perfectly well that even the smallest babies have nerves, but what she *meant* was, that until one has lived long enough and worked hard enough to feel nerve-tired, one has no right even to pretend to be nervous.

Children when really ill can be nervous for a little while, and then every one is sure to be very kind and patient with them. But unless they are very ill, you may be sure that what they call nervousness, is nothing but crossness. They *can* stop crying, or fretting, or fidgeting, if they like, and the sooner they learn to do so, the better for themselves and for everybody else. Any person who gives way to such feelings without real cause, is very weak-minded, and lacks self-control.

The Brain Storehouse

Up in the brain there are a great many little storehouses, in each of which there are many little cells or bottles. In some strange way, every message received is kept in these wee cells. As soon as the servants in the central station receive a message, they bottle it up, and put it away where they can easily find it again.

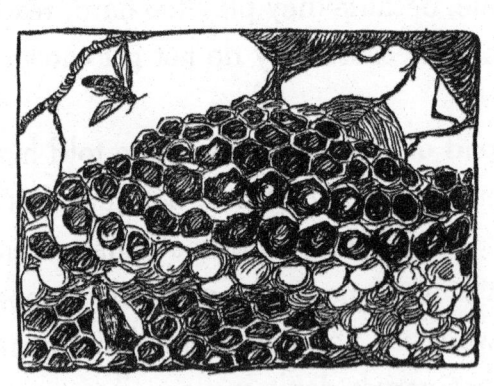

The Brain Has Cells Like a Wasp's Nest—but Much Smaller.

They are such careful servants that they never make any

mistakes. All the messages about form are therefore stored away in one place, all those about color in another, all those about smell in a third, and so it goes on. There is a place for everything in the brain, and everything is in its place.

Let us suppose that the master is sitting up in his office, half asleep, with the shutters of his windows tightly closed. All at once, through the ear nerve close beside him, he hears the one word *"Rose."* "What is rose?" he asks.

Then each of the little servants in turn tells him what is stored up in his "rose cells." The smell servant informs him how nice it smelled, the color servant that it was pink, or red, or white, or yellow, the place servant of the spot where it grew, the feel servant how soft its petals were and how hard its stem. Next, the friendship servant reminds him that it was given to him by some one he loved, the memory servant that he has seen other roses, or that he helped to plant the bush on which it grew, and the worship servant, that the rose was made by God, for the delight of man.

So you see, one word, or one thought, stirs up a big to-do in the brain station; and, whenever the master chooses, his servants will tell him all they know about anything, by bringing out all the information stowed away in their little cells.

GOOD AND BAD STORES

Now we will suppose two little boys playing together. Billy, without meaning to do so hits Johnny. A message flashes up from the place where Johnny was struck, saying: "I am hurt. What shall I do?" Then comes another message from the eyes, saying: "It was Billy who hurt you, I saw him strike you."

When the message servant is asked: "What shall I do?" he does not know, and asks the master. If the master says: "Hit Billy," he quickly sends out a message which makes Johnny's fist strike Billy hard.

Besides, the servant tucks away in the brain storehouse a record of the blow received, and one of the blow given. Now if Johnny is a boy who is always ready to hit back, this servant will find many, many other little cells up in his brain storehouse, packed with the memory of blows.

Then the servant will say to himself: "Ha! every time my master receives a blow, he always says: 'Hit back.' So I do not need to ask him any more what to do. Next time he is struck I'll just send word right away to the fists to strike hard, without troubling him at all about it."

If Johnny said: "Hit back," then thought better of it before his fists could really strike, and made them stop, the message servant records both of these facts. The next time a blow is given, he looks up the two records and is likely to say:

"No; no; I must not send orders to the fists to hit back, because last time master decided that it was best not to strike, although he wanted to do so very badly."

Thus, you see, the little servants, if left to themselves, will be sure to act in the way their master usually wishes. They consult the records, find out what the master generally does, and unless he sends contrary orders, always act in just that way.

When very little I was told that God and the angels saw all that I was doing, and knew all I was saying or thinking. I was also told that the angels kept a big book, in which they wrote down all I said or did, so that they could read it out loud on judgment day. That seemed very wonderful to me.

But what is really more wonderful, is that all our words, all our thoughts, all our actions are kept recorded in our own brain. We may try to forget certain things, but when they are once lodged in one of those wee cells, nothing we can ever do can change them in any way.

Each person bears in his brain a complete record of all he has said, or thought and done. People who think kind thoughts, therefore have their kindness storehouse well stocked, and people who think mean thoughts have the mean storehouse full of horrid messages stored away in their brain.

Our message servants must surely be very sorry, at times, to have to record certain things, and we can imagine one of them, for instance, saying: "See, this is the selfish storehouse. Just look how many cells are stored away here! And each one is full of some selfish deed or thought. I don't like to look at this big supply of selfishness. Over here, in the unselfish storeroom, there are only a very few *small* cells, filled with unselfish deeds and thoughts."

Whenever a message comes up in such a house, saying: "Shall I give up my own will and play the game my sister wishes, or shall I make her play what I wish?" the answer the message servant always sends is: "Make her do as *you* like," unless the master stops it.

Every master should look closely after his storehouses. He cannot pack some of them too full, but there are others which should remain as nearly empty as possible. The storehouses which he should fill up are those of truth, bravery, purity, generosity, unselfishness; and those which should remain empty, are the storehouses where all the bad, greedy, selfish, untruthful, cowardly, mean and dirty words and deeds are stored away.

It is these records—which never lie—which make up what is known as a person's character. A good character is the grandest possession any one can have. All the money, all the genius, all the talent in the world, are not so precious as a good character.

You may work very hard and still never get rich, you may try very hard and yet never get to be a great poet, or musician, or artist, or general, or statesman, or anything else. But you can, if you choose, see that your telegraph servants have none but good deeds and kind words to store away, and thus build up day by day a fine character, the only thing which no one can ever take away from you, and which will be a satisfaction to you forever.

Besides, "It is said there are ten things for which no one has yet been sorry—for doing good to all, for speaking evil of none, for hearing both sides before judging, for thinking before speaking, for holding an angry tongue, for being kind to the distressed, for asking pardon for all wrong, for being patient towards everybody, for stopping the ears to a tale-bearer, for disbelieving all ill reports."

Any one who can train himself to do this is sure to have a fine character in the end.

When a great writer (Walter Scott) was on his deathbed, he said to his son-in-law: "My dear, be a good man, be virtuous—be religious. Be a good man. Nothing else will give you any comfort when you come to lie here."

When people are in sudden danger of death by drowning, fire, or anything of the sort, we are told that all they have done or said, flashes in a moment through their minds. Just think what a relief it must be, when few but good and lovely deeds or words come to stare one in the face when one stands on the brink of eternity.

QUESTIONS.—Which house must you occupy as long as you live, and who is its master? Where are the telephone and telegraph offices in your little house? What are the body telegraph and telephone wires, and where do they run? What bones does the biggest nerve cable string together? Is the master obliged to keep sending orders to his servants or are most of them trained to do their ordinary work without further orders? What does the breathing servant direct; what pleases and what troubles him? Is there a special servant to direct the Pumping Dwarfs, the Stomach Dwarf, etc.? What makes nerves get tired, and how can they get rested? Should sensible children excuse naughtiness by saying, "I'm nervous"? What kind of a storehouse is there in your brain, and what is put away there? Can you mention something good you stored away there to-day? Did you store anything naughty or unkind? If you have many kind, unselfish, gentle stores, what kind of a person will you be? If you store away greedy, selfish, untruthful words and deeds, what kind of a person will you be?

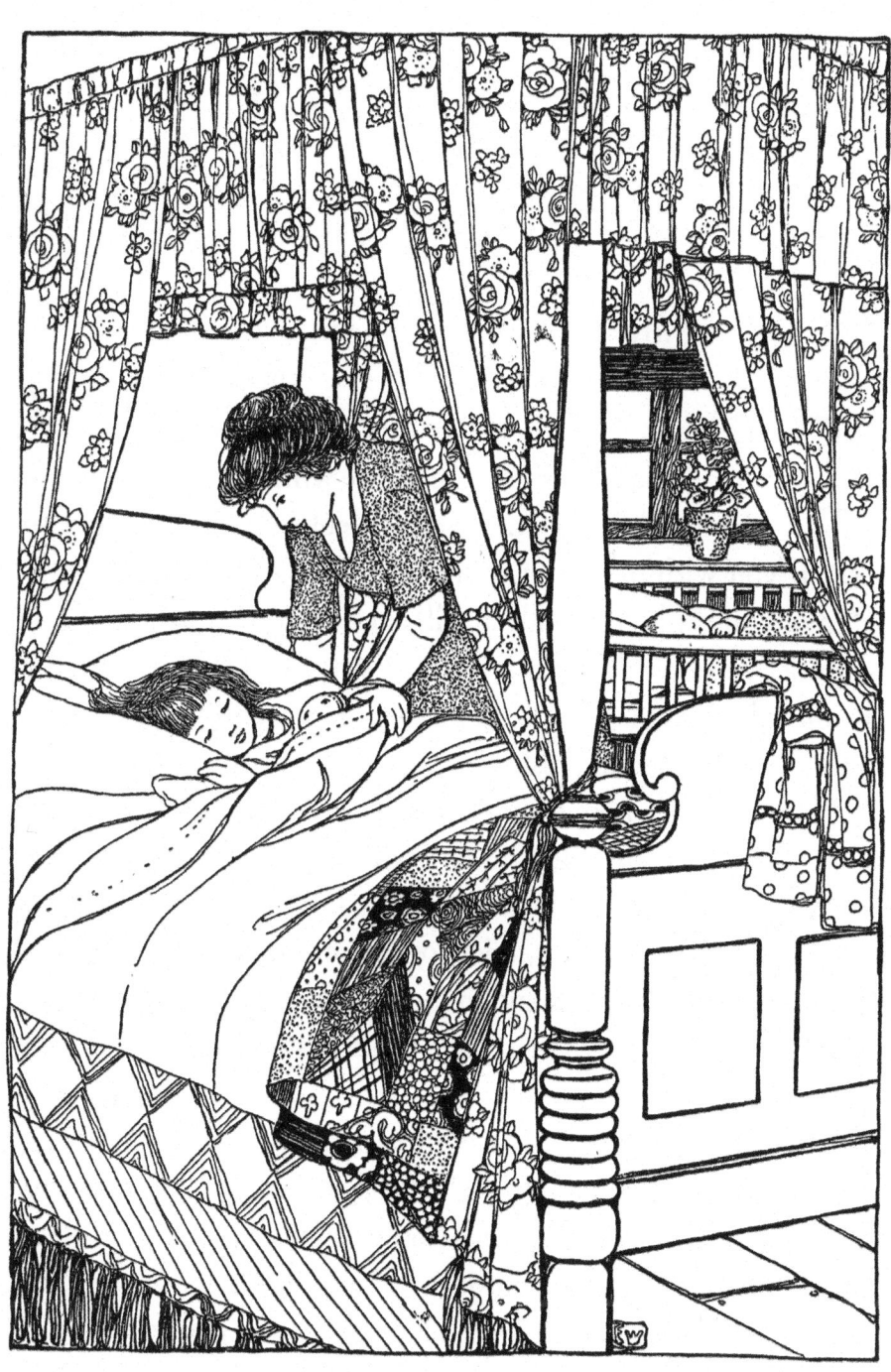

FORM GOOD SLEEPING HABITS

CHAPTER XII

How to Train Body and Mind

THE brain, like all the other parts of our body, needs good food, fresh air (both of which are brought to it by the blood-boats), and plenty of exercise and of rest, if you wish to keep it strong and well. By thinking hard, studying and playing with a will, and by doing everything in a brisk, wide-awake and interested way, you give your brain healthful exercise. By sleeping long and soundly every night, you give it the needed rest.

Wee babies, whose brains are still very weak, and who have everything to learn, sleep a great deal. In fact, they sleep nearly all the time,—which is the very best thing babies can do. Still, as they grow older, and notice more things, they become interested in themselves, and in the world around them, and stay awake for a longer space of time so as to study everything they see.

Almost every baby, if carefully trained from the very first hour of its life, can learn to go to sleep without rocking, singing, or fuss of any kind. He can also be trained very soon to sleep many hours at night without waking up even to be fed. A baby does not, of course, know what he really wants or

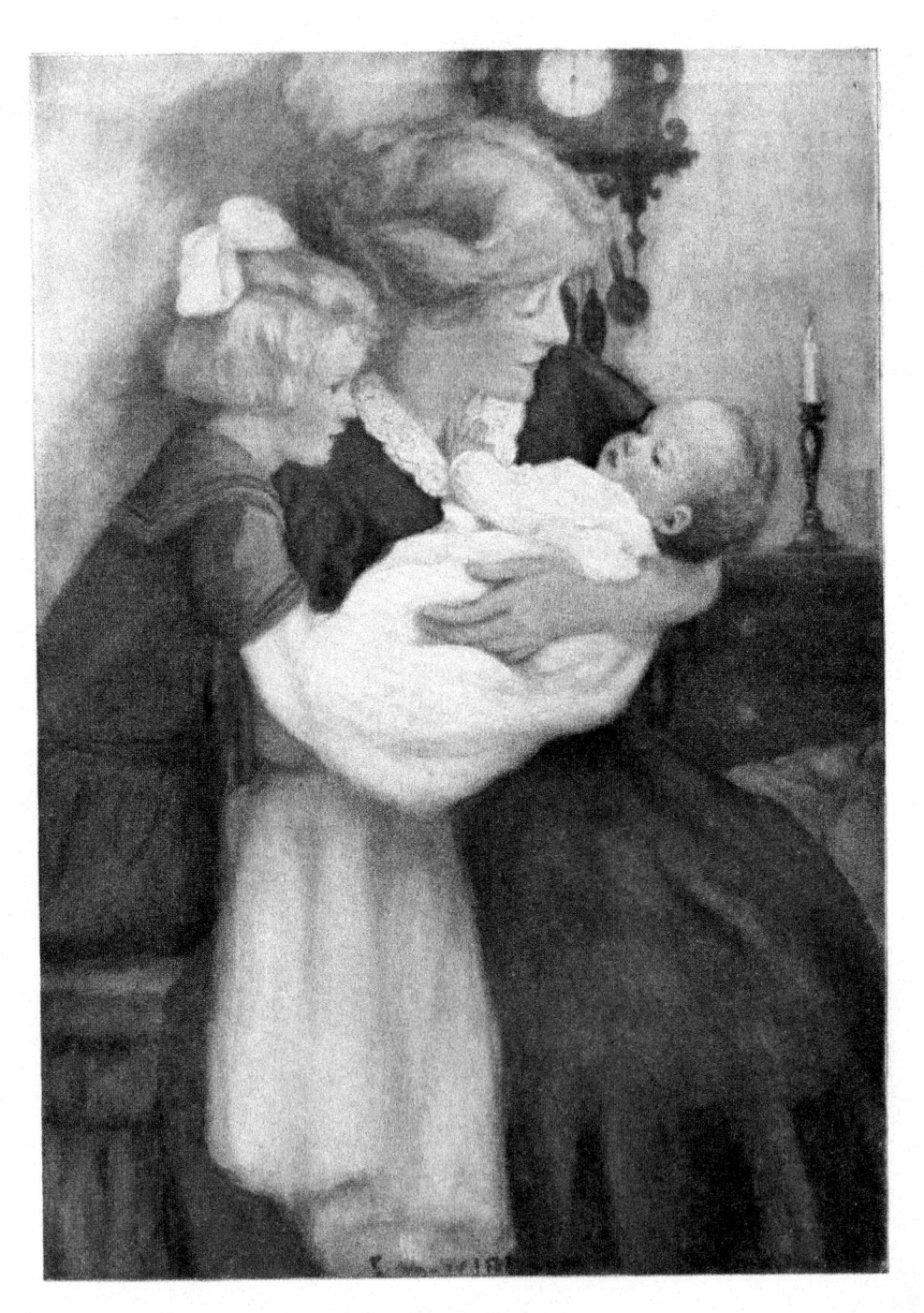

Six O'clock, Bed-time

needs. He is not aware, for instance, of the fact that his little stomach needs a rest between meals. If grown people are not sensible, and feed him every time he wakes up or cries, it will only make him more likely to wake up and cry. Then he will soon turn into a little tyrant, who will make himself and everybody else very unhappy.

By the time a baby is a year old, his waking times are much longer, and his sleeping hours far shorter. Still, he should always go to bed by six o'clock, and stay there twelve or thirteen hours, with very little care or attention during that time, receiving food once or twice only, as the doctor thinks best.

Babies of that age also take two naps every day, one in the morning and one in the afternoon. Until nearly five years of age, every child needs a nap in the daytime, and about twelve hours' sleep at night, if you wish him to keep well and grow strong.

After that, and until ten, a long night rest of twelve or thirteen hours will give him enough sleep. Children between ten and fourteen should always get about eleven hours' rest, and for the next few years, especially if growing fast, nine or ten hours' sleep will not prove a bit too much.

It is far wiser to go to bed at six or eight o'clock and get up early, if you have any studying to do, than to sit up until ten or eleven, and then rise only in time to rush off to school. In fact, most children are far too tired and sleepy to do any studying at all at night; but in the morning, their brains are so rested and bright, that they can learn much faster and better.

If you rise early to study, it is well to drink a glass of milk slowly, and to eat a cracker or piece of bread before you set to work. If you drink your milk fast, or all at once, it is likely to form into a big hard lump in your stomach, and then your little Dwarf will have such a bad time rolling it about, and pulling it to pieces, that it may put him out of temper for the rest of the day.

So be careful of his feelings, and drink your milk slowly. Then, it will form down in your stomach, into many little balls, which your Dwarf can handle very easily, and get rid of long before it is time for the family breakfast.

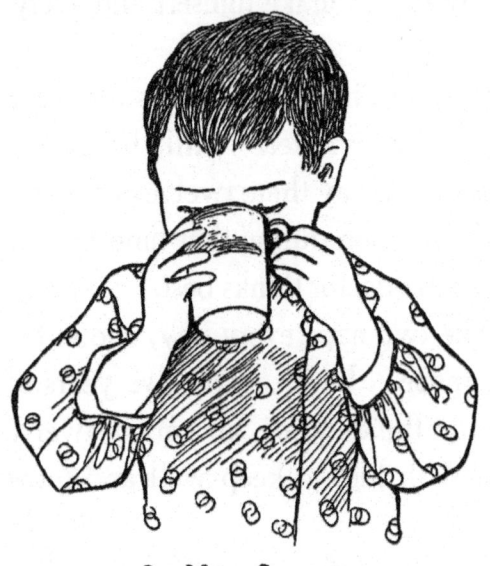

SIP MILK SLOWLY

HOME AFTER DARK

Boys and girls who go to bed *very early* and study in the morning, are much more apt to do good work in school, and to stand well in their classes, than those who sit up late.

Late hours are very bad for children of all ages. Besides that, no child or very young person should ever be out alone after nightfall. Mothers who allow their children to remain out on the street after dark, are really very unkind to them. Sunlight and air are good for everybody, and children should have plenty of play, but *after dark* they should always be gathered in like chickens, close under mother's wing, so that no harm can come to them.

It is much nicer to be at home with father and mother, than wandering around the streets like a stray cat. Mothers who are careful of their children always try to keep them in, but if you have no kind mother to look after you, you should make it a rule to watch yourself, and never to stir away from home after dark.

Girls, in particular, cannot be too careful about this matter. As very bad girls stroll around at night, good girls will surely be mistaken for bad if they are seen out of doors after dark. In fact, no decent woman ever goes out alone after nightfall, unless she has to do so.

In that case, she goes straight about her business, looking neither right nor left, and hurries back home as quickly as she can, so that every one who sees her may know that she is not out for her pleasure, but through necessity. None of you girls should ever pout or be cross when mother insists on your coming in at nightfall, and staying in the house until the next morning. It is the kindest and wisest thing she can do, and instead of grumbling, you ought to put your arms around her neck, and hug her for being so careful of you.

Many a boy and girl has learned evil ways, and gotten into bad habits which ruined a life, merely because allowed to linger out of doors and stroll around for pleasure after dark.

You may be out many times without any harm happening to

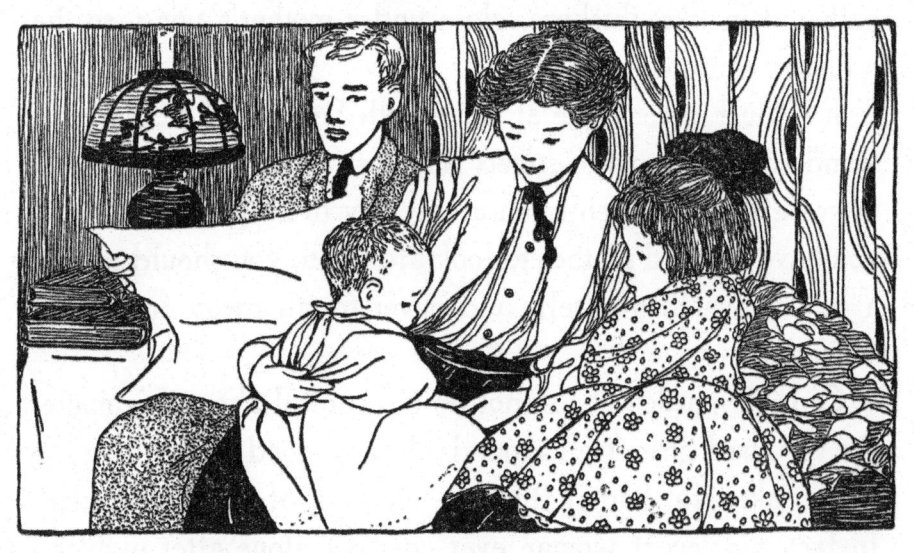

THE BEST WAY TO SPEND EVENINGS.

you, but it is always best to keep on the safe side of things, and in this case that means to learn to be happy and to make others happy in your own home.

I know several large families of boys and girls, who grew up to manhood and womanhood without ever having gone out at night for pleasure, save in the company of their father or mother. These men and women now often say how glad they are that their parents were so strict about this matter, and their hearts are very sore when they see swarms of young people out in the streets at night, and think how sorry all those youngsters will feel, later on, to remember that they spent so many precious hours in that way.

ABOUT BEDS AND BEDDING

If you have eaten just enough plain, wholesome food, drunk pure water, worked and played hard, and done only what is right, you will have no trouble in falling asleep almost as soon as your head touches the pillow, never mind how early you go to bed.

To have a good night's rest, it is often wise not to play or work too hard just before you go to bed. Then, too, make sure that your skin is quite clean, that your night clothes are loose, and that your bed is neatly made.

Next, see that your windows are open in such a way as to supply plenty of fresh air, without the wind blowing in on you, and that there are enough blankets on your bed to keep you just comfortably warm but not too hot.

Lie on your back or side, straightening out your limbs and back, and do not curl up like a dog or a caterpillar. A hard mattress and a thin pillow make the very best kind of a bed for growing boys and girls, each of whom should sleep alone whenever it can be managed.

Doctors tell us that in some strange way, two people sleeping together are very likely to sap one another's strength. An old person sleeping with a child, robs the little one of much of the strength it needs to grow and be happy. When children sleep together, they may not rob each other of so much strength, but they are sure to disturb one another, and not to get as much, or as restful sleep, as if each were alone in his bed.

I know some country children who make their own beds by gathering nice clean corn-husks, drying them carefully, tearing them into narrow strips, and stuffing them into clean bed ticks. This makes fine mattresses, which can be well shaken up every day. Straw in a bed tick, also makes a good mattress, so you see any child can have his own bed at very small cost. Besides, a cot can now be bought for a dollar or less, and any child who is willing to work, can easily earn that much money to buy a bed of his or her own.

In some houses where there are many children, and only very little room, some fathers have cleverly made "double deck beds," such as are seen also in the newsboys' lodging-houses. In this way, each child can sleep alone, and still the bed takes up less floor room than one broad enough for two or more youngsters.

As for baby, a clothes basket padded with cotton batting, and neatly lined with calico that can be washed, makes an excellent bed. One woman I heard about had such a cradle for her baby. By means of a clothes-line, and a few small pulleys screwed into the ceiling, this basket was cleverly swung right over the foot of her bed, so that she could raise it above or lower it down on the bed whenever she pleased.

Thus, if the baby cried or needed anything in the night, the mother stretched out her hand, loosened the rope from its fastenings near the bedhead, and lowered the basket beside her. Then she could reach the baby, without getting up, or catching cold by stepping out of a warm bed on a cold floor. As soon as baby had been cared for, the basket was swung up again, out of reach of all harm, yet not near enough to the ceiling for the child to breathe the bad or hot air which is always found there. Of course, such a cradle is good for a *small* baby only, for when the youngsters begin to climb, it is far better to have a crib for them, with a good strong railing all around it.

LYING ABED MORNINGS

If you don't sleep well, if you have bad dreams, and if you wake up frightened, you may be quite sure it is because you have done something you should not. You have either eaten something which was not good for you, breathed bad air, drunk impure water, worked or played too much or too little, or have been too excited. All you need to do is to watch yourself closely the next day, and if you are wise, and live aright, you will soon sleep soundly all night, and not know a thing until you wake up in the morning.

Some children get in the bad habit of lying abed mornings,

stretching and gaping, and taking another little nap. This is, as we have said, a very bad habit. You should, instead, train yourself to hop right out of bed when you wake up, and not waste any time in the waking process. In fact, a cold water bath is the very best thing to wake any one up very thoroughly.

A great English General (Wellington) used to make his soldiers rise at once when the call sounded, for he always said: "When it is time to turn over, it is time to turn out." Our own great general, George Washington, also believed in doing everything promptly, for when a young officer was tardy one morning, and kept Washington and his staff waiting, he sternly said: "Sir, you may choose to waste your own time, but you have no right to waste ours."

Time spent sleeping is never wasted, provided we have earned the *right* to sleep, and that we *need* rest. But the lazy boy or girl, who drags about from one easy chair to another all day, who neither plays nor studies with any energy, has certainly not earned the right to rest. Still, such children do sleep a great deal, very often, but their sleep does them no good. They crawl slowly out of bed every morning, and are heavy and stupid. Indeed they well deserve the name of "Sleepyhead," which is sure to be given them, and they are not half as nice and attractive as the wideawake youngsters, who are busy all day and sleep "like tops" all night.

The harder you work, the more you deserve and the more you need a good night's rest. Sleep will give your tired brain a chance to rest, and while you are thus lost to everything, your blood-boats can go on carrying material to your weary muscles and nerves, so that they too can make up for the loss of the day, and be strong and fresh when you again need them on the morrow.

If you make the best use of your waking hours, you can surely get all the needful work done without robbing yourself of any sleep. Besides, that kind of a theft is sure to do you a great deal of harm. People who *won't* sleep, *can't* sleep after awhile, even when they wish to do so, and if one does not get sleep enough, one is sure to feel ill, and perhaps in time to become crazy.

THE WAY TO STUDY

I have seen children open their books to study, think one minute of their lesson, look around the next to see what mother is doing, then read a word or two, listen to what father is saying, stare out of the window, and only come back to the lesson every once in a while.

It takes such youngsters a very long time to learn even the simplest thing, and then they only half know it. But, if they put all their minds on their lesson, thought of that, and that only, tried hard to understand just what it meant, and to fix it firmly in their minds, it would soon be packed away safely in the brain storehouse, and the memory servant would bring it out perfectly clear whenever the master chose to call for it. A few *minutes* of intent work is far better than *hours* of dawdling study.

There was once a poor boy, named Elihu Burritt. He had to earn his living by blowing the bellows for a cross blacksmith. This boy was very eager to learn and as he could not afford to buy books,—which were very costly in his day,—he borrowed all he could.

As he had no time or place to sit down and read comfortably, he used to prop these books, wide open, on a beam just over his bellows. Every time he raised his hand to grasp the handle of the bellows, he read as many words as he could catch in that glance. Then he would think hard of these words, while hanging on to the bellows' handle, which had to be forced down by his weight. When he rose again, the lad read the next few words, and he went on so, until he had finished page after page, and book after book.

By making such good use of these few seconds between every pull of his bellows, this brave boy not only managed to educate himself well, but learned to read many different languages, and became one of the most learned men in the world.

You see, he trained his eye to be quick and find the place where he left off reading, his memory to receive a thing which he had seen only once, and his mind to think hard about whatever he read.

Most boys, placed as he was, would have declared that they had no time to study, for they had to work hard all day;

but this one knew that a few minutes at a time, given every day to any study, with the firm resolve to do one's best, are bound to bring about great results in the end.

Do not wait, therefore, until you have plenty of time to begin anything. Begin now. Use all the little odds and ends of time you have, learn to do things in such a way as to *save* time, and before long you will find out that you have leisure enough to do many things if you only choose to do them.

THE SENSES

Man has five senses as they are called. These are the means by which he can see, hear, smell, taste and touch. Most of us have all these senses complete, but a few poor children are deaf, or blind, or without any sense of smell or taste. Children who have not the use of all five senses miss a great deal of the good we have to enjoy, and we should, therefore, be very kind to them and try to help them in any way we can.

You all know that we see by means of our eyes, which we have called until now the windows of our little houses. But eyes are much more than windows. I suppose most of you children have seen a camera, with which photographs are taken. Well, our eyes are the finest and best cameras ever made.

Every picture which passes in front of those windows, when the curtains (eyelids) are raised, is quickly photographed.

The photograph servant—who, we will make believe lives there—takes one snap-shot after another, and then his helpers stow all these photographs away in the brain storehouse, where the master can call for them whenever he pleases, and look them all over as often as he likes.

If we look at pleasant people and beautiful things, we have many lovely pictures to stow away in our private picture gallery, but if we look at cross people and hateful things, we have pictures which can give us no pleasure to look over later on.

These wonderful cameras of ours are very delicate. As we have only two of them, and cannot get new ones when these are out of order or worn out, we must take very good care of them. To take the best care of your eyes, you should always keep them clean, never rub or touch them with dirty fingers, and work or study only when the light is good and when you are not tired.

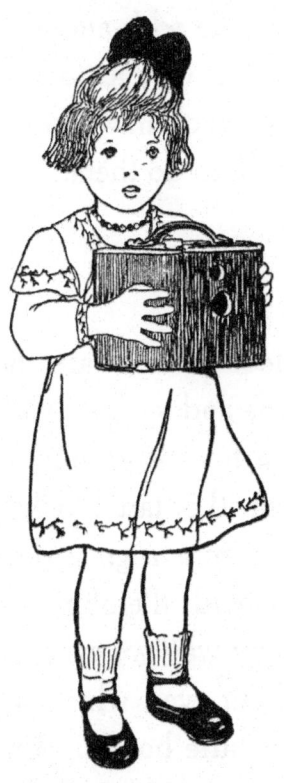

THE EYES ARE LIKE A CAMERA

If you read or sew when it grows dark, when the light is dim, when the sun is shining brightly on your book or work, or when you are tired, you are likely to strain your eyes. Never try to look hard at very bright objects—like the sun,—and do not strain your eyes or tire them in any way.

If you cannot see well, you should have your eyes examined, and wear glasses, so that your eyes may be helped to do you as good service as they can for as long a time as possible.

Baby's eyes need special care if you wish him to see well when he grows up. So be very careful not to let the sun shine right into them when he is in his carriage, and place the light where it cannot fall upon him when he is asleep.

Besides that, you should keep baby's eyes clean, by washing them carefully every day. Eyes are so delicate that they must be bathed very, very gently, but plenty of water is good for them at all times. If they feel tired, it is often good to give them an extra washing, with water as hot as you can bear it.

One can also train one's eyes to see more or less quickly all that one wishes them to take in. Deaf mute children whom I know, can glance at pictures and take in every detail in a flash. They often surprise me because they see and think so well. Those children have learned to *see* what their friends say by watching their lips. You see they are making good use of their eyes! They learn to talk by imitating the motions of other people and feeling how they use the muscles of their throats.

About Hearing

Blind children learn mostly by hearing and by touch. Their sense of touch is so very quick and so delicate, that they can read raised print as fast and as well as other children can read ordinary print. Some children, who are blind and deaf, like Helen Keller, for instance, are obliged to learn nearly everything by means of touch alone.

This brave girl worked and worked, until at sixteen she knew enough to enter college, passing the same examinations as older girls, who could both see and hear, and getting high marks, too!

In college she studied so faithfully that she won her diploma, like the girls who could see and hear. She then decided to spend her life in helping the blind, deaf, and dumb and is now leading a busy useful life. I am sure you will never hear of a brighter or braver girl, or one who deserves more praise for being always cheerful, hopeful and busy in spite of her great trials.

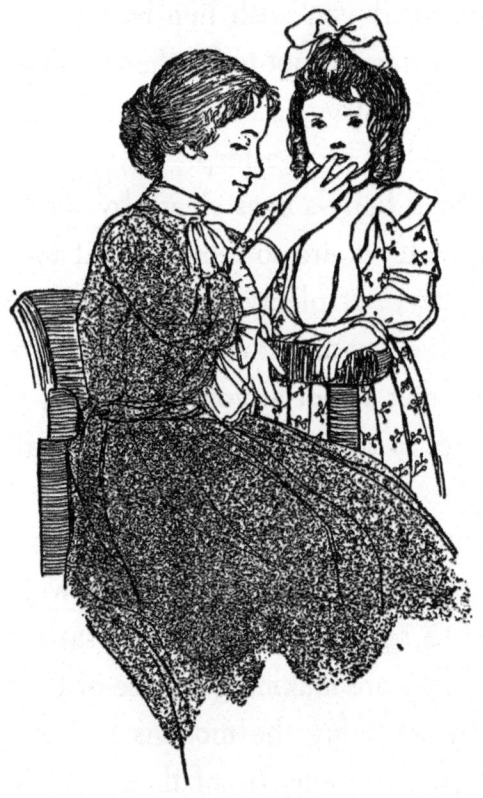

HEARING BY TOUCH

We, who have all our senses, ought not only to be very thankful, but to see that we make the very best use of them. They were given us to use, for good or evil just as we choose, but if we only make good use of them we know we will be a blessing to ourselves and to everybody else.

Besides training our eyes to see good things, to like those best, and to dwell as little as possible on those which are really ugly or hateful, we can teach our ears to love beautiful sounds and to hear by preference all that is good. The ears you know, are the telephones of our little house. Any one can call up anything he pleases through an ear-telephone, which receives all kinds of messages.

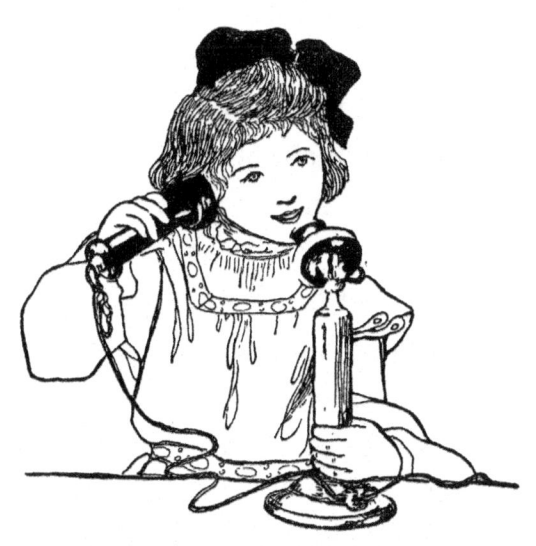

THE EAR IS A SORT OF TELEPHONE

But, the master can heed these or not, just as he pleases, and a wise master listens only to what is good and right.

Whenever anything wrong or unpleasant is being said, he quickly sends a message down to the hands, bidding them close the openings to the ear-telephone, so that no more of the talk that he does not like shall come up into the station to be stowed away in his brain.

I would advise all children to stop up their ears tight, in this way, whenever any one says anything which they feel is not right, and to run away, for they surely do not want their brain storehouse all filled up with memories of bad words, evil suggestions, naughty or unkind speeches or mean thoughts!

Our ears, like our eyes, are very delicate indeed. They, too, need to be kept quite clean, by frequent and careful washings. Never poke anything into your ears, save the tip of your finger or a corner of your sponge, wash-cloth, or handkerchief, and be sure that nature will take care of any wax which you cannot reach in that way.

Keep your ears clean, do not let a sharp draught blow into them, try not to let them get too cold, and if they ache, never use anything but hot water, hot cloths, or a few drops of sweet oil heated in a spoon and carefully dropped into the hole. If this does not cure your earache, it will be best for you to see a doctor, because the ears and eyes are very delicate and precious and nobody can afford to neglect them. If you are too poor to pay a doctor, you know you can always go to the nearest hospital, where you will be taken care of, and where they will give you medicine and advice free of charge.

QUESTIONS.—How can you exercise and how can you rest your brain? How much sleep should babies have, and how much is best for you? What is the best time to study, early in the morning, or late at night, and why? Why should you drink milk slowly? Where is the best place for boys and girls after dark? What is the best kind of a bed for growing children? If you don't sleep well, and have bad dreams, what is the matter? Is it right to lie abed late, or should one rise right away when called? Describe two ways of studying; which is better? Could you

About Hearing 195

tell how Elihu Burritt got his education? How many senses have you; what are they called, and what do they do? What kind of pictures can you pack away in your brain store-house? How should you take care of your eyes and what kind of a light should you have when you wish to read or sew? If any talk is going on around you, which you should not hear, what order should the house-master send to the hands and feet?

CHAPTER XIII

GOOD AND BAD DRINKING HABITS

YOU all like fairy tales, do you not? Well, nearly everybody has liked them at some time in his life, and in olden times many people believed that fairy tales were quite true. They thought, for instance, that somewhere in the world there was a wonderful fountain, and that if one could only drink of its waters and bathe in them, one would become young and strong, and remain so forever after.

The belief in the "Fountain of Youth" was so great, that many men spent their lives seeking for it, and when they failed to find it in Europe, some of them even came over to America in the vain hope of discovering it here at last.

Other men fancied that it was possible to find a Water of Life, or a medicine which would make an old man feel young again, and would prevent his ever dying. They began to mix and boil all sorts of drugs and drinks, and finally one of them, by accident, found out the way to make brandy or distilled liquor. He tasted it and when his cheeks flushed, his body grew warm, and he felt like singing and dancing, he thought he had surely found what he sought. He gave some of it to his friends, who also felt very young and lively when they had drunk

Good and Bad Drinking Habits

it, and all declared that the Water of Life was found!

For many, many years people believed as he did, that those who drank of the Water of Life would live forever. But soon they found out their mistake, for the warmth and feeling of jollity lasted only a short time, and they had to drink more and more of the liquor to feel any good effects from it.

By and by some died who had drunk most freely of the Water of Life. And then every one knew that the new discovery was a fraud! Still, many people *liked* the taste of it, *enjoyed* the feeling of warmth and merriment which it aroused, and *thought* that it did them much good. They said that although the liquor could not make one *live* forever, it gave new strength and spirits, and could cure all manner of diseases.

This belief,—which has caused much sorrow, as you will see,—was all wrong, but it spread and spread, until almost everywhere men called for drinks containing more or less of the so-called Water of Life, which, had it been rightly named, would have been called the Water of Death. The drink which caused the feelings I have described, was really harmful and it is the same which we now call alcohol.

As the real Water of Life was very costly, some men soon found out ways of making cheap imitations, and other less costly drinks, which contained a small part of the same mixture, and therefore satisfied the taste of those who clamored for it.

These drinks are now made and sold everywhere, and although some time ago people began to find out that they were very bad indeed for most human beings, they still are used everywhere and millions of dollars are spent for them in our country every year.

Even doctors were long cheated by these drinks, which contained alcohol, for they noticed that the heart beat faster, the skin flushed, and that new strength and courage seemed to enter into the people to whom they gave it. Still, little by little they learned that while it *seemed* to do good for a few minutes, it really did well people a great deal of harm, and also injured the sick in many cases.

They discovered that all drinks which contain any alcohol act just like a whip. You know that when you whip up a tired horse, he will make a new effort; but whipping does not add one bit to his strength, and the new effort he makes only results in exhausting him sooner and more completely.

The Yeast Plant

As I said before, it was a long, long time before even the wisest doctors began to suspect that alcohol was mostly a cheat and generally harmful. Meantime, many other doctors, and countless men and women, praised it, sang about it, wrote poems upon it, and drank it freely whenever they chose.

In fact, some kind of liquor was always offered wherever you went, and you were considered rude if you did not drink it. At marriages, christenings, burials, at church raisings, balls, and dinners, people drank, and there was a time when some even prided themselves upon the amount they could drink without falling down under the table, dead drunk.

While they, in their ignorance, were acting thus, other wise people were little by little finding out all they could about the evil effects of alcohol, and trying to show how wrong it is to ruin one's health by touching it in any form.

After much study and many experiments,—for they really *wanted* to find that it was something else, and not alcohol which was at the root of all the harm—wise men discovered, as I tell you, that any drink which contains the least drop of alcohol is bad for human beings in general, and that, it is after all nothing but a cheat.

They found out that when you squeeze grapes, or apples, or any other kind of fruit, you get some juice which contains more or less sugar, because most fruits are sweet. Clinging to the skin of the fruit thus squeezed, and floating around in the air we breathe, there are many, many little seeds of what is called the yeast plant. When these fall into the fruit juice, they begin to grow, and as they grow they change much of the sugar into alcohol. Then the juice bubbles and boils over the jug in which it is kept, just as if a fire, which you cannot see, were made under it. Still, the fruit juice never gets really hot, although its taste and nature change entirely.

Because apples and grapes are good for people, many men will tell you that wine and cider can do no harm. But a very few hours after the juice has been squeezed out of these fruits, we know that the little yeast plant has begun its evil work, and that it is busy changing the sugar—the food part of fruit—into something quite different, which is not food at all, and which is really a kind of poison.

Beer and ale are made from grain. The starch of the grain is first changed into sugar, then the yeast plant sets to work to make the sugar into alcohol. People will tell you that as beer and ale are made from grain, you have all the strength of the grain in liquid form. This is not true. By careful study and experiment, it has been found out that there is more real food and strength contained in the flour which you can hold on the point of your knife blade, than in eight quarts of the best beer that was ever made!

Although people found out that alcohol was harmful some time ago, only a few were willing to believe it, and even those few little suspected what very bad effects could come from using it, and that it was to be found in so many things.

You will, no doubt, be greatly surprised when I tell you that there is a great deal of alcohol in every loaf of bread which is ready to be put into the oven. The alcohol gets into the bread by means of the yeast, which is put into it to make it light.

When the bread is put into the oven, the alcohol gets very hot and flies off in steam. In getting out of the bread it makes some of the little holes which we can see, and which make good bread so light and spongy. All the alcohol in a loaf of bread has been turned to steam, and has gone out of it even before it is entirely baked, and as no taste of it is left in our bread, we can eat it without any fear of harm.

HARMFUL DRINKS

Some good women, who know how bad alcohol is for everybody, often make currant wine and root beer. Because they make it themselves, and do not put any alcohol in it, they will tell you in all good faith: "You can drink that without fear. There is not a drop of alcohol in it. I made it myself, and I can answer for it that it is a harmless drink."

The poor souls are, however, sorely mistaken. Unless they boiled the juice hard and bottled it up, right away, in air-tight bottles, they *could not* keep the yeast plant out of it, or prevent its growing and changing the sugar in their wine or beer into alcohol.

Even when making preserves, and screwing them up into air-tight jars, you cannot quite be sure of shutting out all yeast plant seeds. That some do slip in at times, is proved by the fact that the fruit in our jars sometimes ferments, and that when you want to use it you often find it spoiled.

There is alcohol in nearly every kind of drink, and wherever there is alcohol there is danger. Alcohol never does *well* people any good, and it does a great deal of harm to nearly every one who makes a habit of drinking it.

The only drinks in which no alcohol, or other harmful things can be found, and which are really safe in every way,

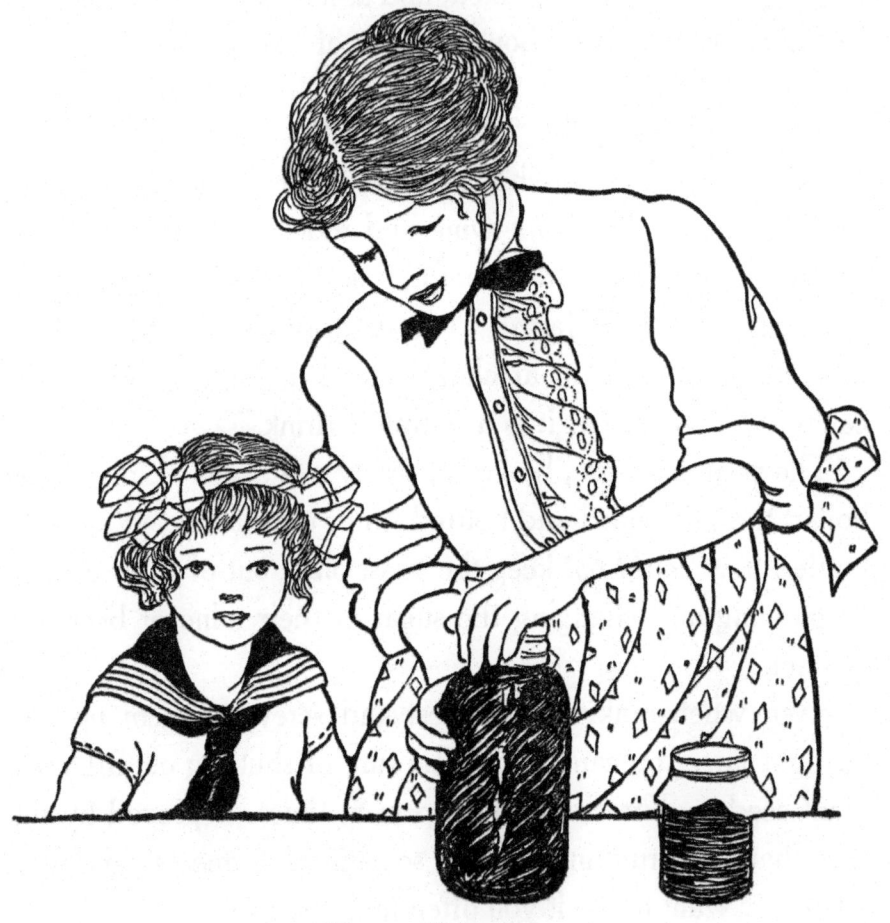

MAKING PRESERVES

are pure water, milk and not too sweet lemonade. Surely those are enough to quench the thirst of any reasonable boy or girl. There are many other drinks which are only a *little* hurtful, so little that it hardly matters, but brandy, whisky, rum, gin, ginger-ale, ale, beer, root beer, and all kinds of wines and liquors are sure to contain more or less alcohol, even if those who sell them neither know—nor wish you to know,—how much of that stuff is to be found in them.

THE HARM ALCOHOL DOES

Some of you may wonder what harm alcohol does, so I will try to explain so that you will be sure to understand.

A man was once wounded in such a way that he had a hole in his body, through which the doctors could look right into his stomach and find out just what was going on inside there. They saw that every time this man drank anything containing alcohol, his stomach got very red and sore looking, and stayed so a long time.

You see, alcohol is a drink, so strong, that it burns and stings the delicate skin of the mouth, the food tube, and the stomach.

Alcohol itself does not stay in the stomach long, but is soon sucked up by the little tubes, and carried off to the liver. The Liver Dwarf hates it, because it makes all *his* tubes red and sore, and after a while it hardens them so they can do no more good work.

As the liver cannot do anything with alcohol, it has to pass on into the blood. When it gets to the heart, the Pumping Dwarfs—who also hate alcohol—pull their ropes quicker and quicker to get rid of the blood-boats loaded with it.

The blood then rushes to all parts of the body, where alcohol makes all the tubes red and sore, but where it does no good at all. When the blood-boats reach the little canals near the surface, the red shows right through the skin of the person who has been drinking, who therefore looks very flushed.

When the little blood-boats laden with alcohol, reach the brain, the worst mischief begins. As the brain is the most delicate part of the body, it suffers most when the blood, which is sent to feed it, does not contain the right kind of food, or brings anything which can hurt it.

Alcohol is so strong and so biting, that when it reaches the brain, it makes the reason servant dead drunk, and he does not try any longer to restrain the laughing servant, the crying servant, or the talking servant, all of whom begin acting just as they please.

I am afraid that all of you, at some time, have seen drunken men. Well, you know that at first they are very jolly, talk, and laugh aloud, and act very foolishly. But by and by—when the blood-boats have brought still more alcohol into the poor delicate brain,—the servant who sends out all the messages about walking, standing and moving is also overcome by the alcohol. It is then a man begins to stagger and wobble, and finally falls down in a heap, dead drunk.

When the blood-boats bring enough alcohol to stun nearly all the servants up in the brain, and to put the master himself sound asleep, the body lies like a log. The drunken man breathes heavily, and stays in a stupor, until his skin, lungs and kidneys, can manage to drive enough alcohol out of the body, so that his servants can little by little recover their senses, and set to work again.

But the servants are all very cross after alcohol has thus made them stupid and sleepy. They move slowly and uncertainly, and feel sick and so tired that they do their work very badly indeed. In fact, alcohol stays a long time in the body, making mischief. It has even been found that it takes from three to six days to get quite rid of the alcohol in one bottle of beer only, and still beer contains only a little that is harmful compared to many other drinks.

Why People Drink

As you have already seen, drink does harm to all the parts of the body, but you have as yet heard of only a small part of the damage it really does.

One glass of liquor may cause as many as eight thousand extra heart beats before the blood-boats can carry it away. Of course, so much extra work must make the Pumping Dwarfs tired and sore, especially as they dislike alcohol very much indeed.

If the heart beats eight thousand times more than usual for *one* glass of liquor, just imagine how many times extra the poor thing has to thump when many drinks are taken each and every day. No wonder that life insurance companies count that a man of twenty, who drinks, will not live much longer than thirty-five, while a man of twenty, who does not drink, will live to be sixty-five at least.

As drunken men do not know what they are doing, they often give away all they have, or allow others to steal it; thus they ruin their families as well as their own health. Besides, a man who drinks, soon passes from the talkative, jolly stage of feeling, into a state of blind fury with everybody and everything. In this state, men—who when they were sober, were kind and good—have become like wild animals, and have committed awful crimes.

Such are the bad effects of drink, that those who know, will tell you that seven-tenths of all the poverty and crime in the United States is due to alcohol. Still, in spite of this, and of the fact that they know it hurts them, many men will go on drinking. Some drink because they like the taste of the liquor, some because they are weak-minded, and cannot resist when any one makes fun of them for being afraid of it, and some because by drinking they have become the victims of the drink disease, and cannot stop themselves any more.

Those who just *like* the taste of alcohol, or who drink it merely because they wish to do as their friends do, are self-indulgent, weak-minded fools. They are probably men,—or women alas,—who, when young children, were either indulged or neglected, and who never did anything except what they liked, and because it pleased or suited them to do it.

They have no real idea of duty or self-control, and they are without character. When they were young, every time a message came up to the telegraph servant, their answer always was: "Do that because it pleases me." The result was that the selfish, self-indulgent storehouse had many new cells stowed away in it every day. After a while, the servant, said: "Oh, my master thinks of himself only, and always does as he likes best, regardless of the feelings or rights of others. It is no use even to *ask* what he wants me to do. I know it already." Then the servant sent out new messages, ordering the taste to please itself, and thus more cells were added to the self-indulgent storehouse.

If the master drinks because he is a coward, and dares not say "No," even when he knows it would be right to do so, new cells are daily added to the storehouse where all the cowardly deeds are bottled up, and the man sinks lower and lower in everybody's esteem.

Such a person can stop drinking any moment the master in his little house really makes up his mind not to do it any more. But the servants have so thoroughly learned bad habits that they will have to be watched very closely if he wishes to reform. Every time a message comes: "Here is a glass of liquor, what is to be done with it?" these servants,—unless the master interferes quickly and decidedly—will answer back:

"Drink it, of course. That is what master always orders. There are any number of cells here saying 'Drink,' and hardly any at all saying, 'Don't drink.'"

You see, do you not, how very watchful such a master has to be to prevent his servants acting in the usual way before he can stop them. But, after he has stopped them many, many times, and when the "Don't drink" cells get to be more and more numerous in his brain storehouse, the servant is no longer in such a hurry to answer: "Master always pleases his taste," or "Master is afraid to say no," and says instead: "Just wait a minute, and I'll find out what master wishes this time. There are so many cells up here which say 'Drink' and so many which say 'Don't drink,' that I am quite bewildered, and don't know any more what to do."

Thus, any person *can* get rid of a bad habit. But it is far, far easier never to get into bad habits at all. If a house master, from the very first, always directs his servants never to touch drink because it is bad for the body, there will be no "drink cells" at all in his brain storehouse, and after a while his servants will answer all such messages themselves saying: "Oh! take that stuff away, for master knows far better than ever to drink a drop of it."

Why You Should Not Drink

Some men have brains built in such a way that the very least little drop of alcohol is not only bad for them, but may start a terrible disease. Sometimes their brains can more easily take this awful disease because their father or mother, or even their grandfather or grandmother, used to drink.

You all know that you have mouths, eyes, noses, hair or some other feature like your father or mother. Well, just as some parts of the outside of your body are exact copies of the same parts of one of your parents, some of the inside parts of your body are like theirs too.

A man who drinks, and who has "drink cells" in his brain storehouse, is most likely to have children, whose storehouses seem just aching to get full of "drink cells" too. If such children drink once, because they "want to know what it tastes like," or because "one little drink cannot do me any harm," they *begin* storing away "drink cells," and so perhaps give that bad disease the very chance it was seeking to start and grow and take such a strong hold upon them that it will never let them go again.

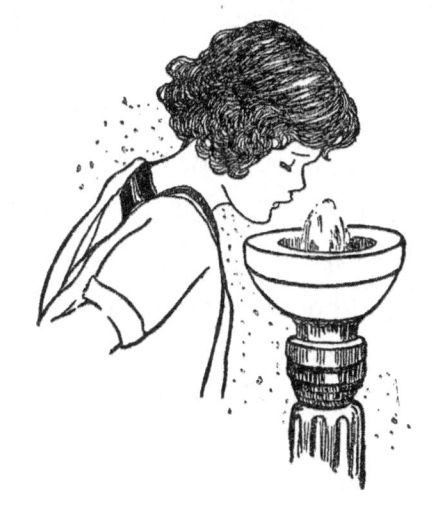

A SAFE DRINK

Children whose p a r e n t s drink, therefore, should be very, very careful never to touch any kind of liquor, however mild. To strengthen their brains they should eat wholesome food, breathe fresh air, take plenty of exercise, keep clean, and train their bodies and minds in every way to do only that which is right and noble. If they begin early, if they try very hard, and if they never give in, or never give up trying to get into good habits, such children will make the finest and best men and women in our country; men and women whom every one will respect, and whom all will admire and try to imitate. They will deserve much more credit for being good, and never yielding to the temptation to drink, than any of the people who never have to struggle against such a temptation.

There are many people who laugh and joke when they see a man stagger along under the influence of drink, or talk and act foolishly. Then there are some who make others drunk just to see what they will say or do. The people who laugh are thoughtless, or heartless, and those who make others do wrong for fun are wicked. Now, it is not right to be even thoughtless, for every one should feel it a duty to help and encourage his neighbor to do only that which is right and good.

There are some very good people who think that all drunkards are equally vile. These people evidently do not know, or they will not believe, that while some drinkers are only weak and evil-minded others are really very ill with a disease, which, when once it has taken hold of them, they can no longer resist.

Doctors, who know about the drink disease, despise the men who drink merely because the liquor *tastes* good, but pity the poor men who drink because they are victims of this awful sickness. Most diseases can be cured, however, if rightly treated and in time, and many a drunkard could be saved, if his family and friends only knew what to do, and were willing to do it with all their might.

If you ever wish to help cure a person with this drink disease, you should see that he is kept warm and comfortable, that he has plenty of sleep and exercise, fresh air in abundance, a really clean skin, plain food nicely cooked, and that his thoughts are made to dwell on good things only, as much as possible.

Such a man needs to be watched as closely as a crazy man, so that he does not harm himself by drinking. Just as crazy men often have to be shut up in asylums for the insane, these drunken men often have to be locked up in asylums, where they take care of people suffering from the drink disease, and try to cure them of their terrible trouble.

STRONGER WITHOUT THAN WITH LIQUOR

It is because drink does such fearful harm to many people, that there are laws in our country saying when, where and how liquor can be sold. In some places, where the voters have at last realized the harm that liquor can do, there are also laws forbidding the sale of all drinks in which alcohol can be found. When you get old enough to vote, or to influence those who do vote, perhaps you will try to stop the sale of liquor, as much as you can, so that the terrible drink disease shall spread no further, and our country go to pieces as all the countries have done in turn where wrong-doing was not stopped for good and all.

When few or no drunkards shall be left on the globe, much of the unhappiness will be ended, there will be far less crime, and much less sickness. Doctors tell us that seven out of every ten sick people in the city hospitals are ill, only because they or their parents drank, or because they were hurt by people who were drunk. There is in one part of New York City, a saloon for every fifty-eight persons, and a school for every sixty-six thousand. Do you think that can be good for the people or for the city? If you could vote would you not vote to have that changed?

Until now, in speaking of drink we have talked about drunkards only. But there are ever and ever so many men and women, who never were drunk in their lives, who only drink a very little, and who do not know or believe that even a little alcohol, in any form, can do them or their children any harm. Some say: "You see I am far from strong, so I have to take a little wine or beer to give me strength."

If they only knew it, the wine or beer does not give them any strength at all. Of course, there was a time when everybody thought it did, but now a few people know better. There are clever machines which measure people's strength. Men who said they drank because liquor made them stronger, have been tested by these machines. They were tried when they had not taken a drop of any kind of liquor for many, many days, and when they themselves said that they had no strength at all. Then they were tried again when they had taken some liquor, and said they felt much stronger and were sure they could do much better.

Strange to relate, the machines proved that they were really much stronger when they had not drunk and *felt* weak, than when they had drunk and *felt* strong. It is in this way that doctors have proved that drink is a cheat, and that it does not give well people the strength that so many of them suppose.

Another proof that liquor does not give strength is the fact that college-teams are never allowed to touch a single drop of it, while the men are training for their great matches. Don't you suppose the trainers would *make* them drink if there was any chance that alcohol would make them stronger?

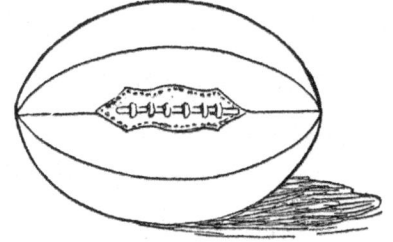

FOOT-BALL PLAYERS MUST NOT TOUCH LIQUOR

During the Spanish-American war our sailors were not allowed to have any liquor when about to fight, while the Spaniards received their usual allowance. The result was that our men won victory after victory, lost no ships and very few lives, while the Spaniards were beaten, lost all their ships, and ever so many of their men.

About Temperance

Some men say that they must drink to keep warm, especially when they are going out in the cold. They are sorely mistaken in thinking that drink will make or keep them warm. Drink will only drive more hot blood near their skin, where they can feel it, but where the cold air will strike and cool it off sooner. Then it will go back to the heart much cooler than it was before.

In Russia, where it is very cold, we are told that the officers, who have to go out with the troops, smell the breath of every man before they start. Any man whose breath shows that he has been drinking, is sent right back to camp or to the barracks, for the officers know that he will be the first to be overcome by the cold, and the most likely to be frost-bitten or frozen to death.

When explorers go far north, or south, on journeys of discovery, trying to reach the north or south pole, they no longer drink themselves, or allow their men to drink, because they have found that the only way to keep the body warm enough is *not* to drink liquor of any kind.

Some engineers were surveying in South America, and climbed a very high mountain. They reached a place where the snow never melts, even in the hottest summers, for the higher you go the colder it gets.

These engineers had to spend the night up there, amid snow

and ice. Some of them drank a great deal of liquor "to keep warm," others drank a little "to take the chill off," but a few of the men were wise enough not to drink at all. When morning came, those who drank a great deal were dead—frozen stiff,—those who drank a little, had badly frost-bitten hands and feet; while those who had not touched liquor at all were alive and well, ready to bury or nurse the others.

In hot countries it is equally dangerous to drink, and during the many wars in Africa, the generals who have been most successful are those who neither drank themselves nor allowed their men to drink. In fact it is now clearly shown that *well* people do not need liquor at any time, because it cannot really help them in any way. On the contrary, it always does them some harm, although many of them do not realize that the troubles they have often come from drink only.

Still, as long as people want liquor of any kind, it will be made and sold. Because liquor does harm and causes much sin and unhappiness many of the temperance people say that all those who make and sell it are very wicked men. This is not quite true.

Many makers and sellers of liquor never touch it themselves, and teach their children to leave it alone; but they say that as long as people *will* have it, it is far better that they should make and sell it, because *they* at least will give the people the best liquor that can be made.

Many of these men did not know when they were boys that

liquor could do any harm unless too much of it was taken, for if you drink too much water or too much milk, you can harm your health too. Temperance really means just enough of anything and no more.

A man, who when a boy, always heard that there was no harm at all in dealing in liquor, or even drinking a little of it, has this idea so deeply rooted in his brain, that it is not likely any one can ever change it.

Many of us think that if most of the men who make liquor, who sell it, and who drink it, had only been told, when boys, just what it is and what harm it can do, they would never have touched it at all, and would certainly have chosen another way of making their living.

You boys, who read such books as this, and who are taught in school while you are young, all the harm that alcohol can do, will, therefore, be greatly to blame, if, when you grow up and can do as you please, you ever drink, or help to make or to sell any of the drinks which have caused so much sin, sorrow and shame in this world.

The Use of Alcohol

You have already heard all the bad about alcohol that I care to tell you. Now I am going to tell you some good about it, and there is really a great deal of good to say. It is not the fault of poor alcohol itself, if some men have made and still make bad use of it.

Alcohol is just splendid to burn. It makes a nice clear flame without any smoke at all. If you put it in a lamp, and hang a small kettle over the flames, you can have boiling water in a very short time, and the bottom of your kettle will be quite clean when you are through using it.

When you have sick people in the house, or when you want to heat baby's food at night, an alcohol lamp is often very convenient. Besides, dentists, jewelers, and many other skilled workmen are very glad indeed to use alcohol lamps for much of their fine work.

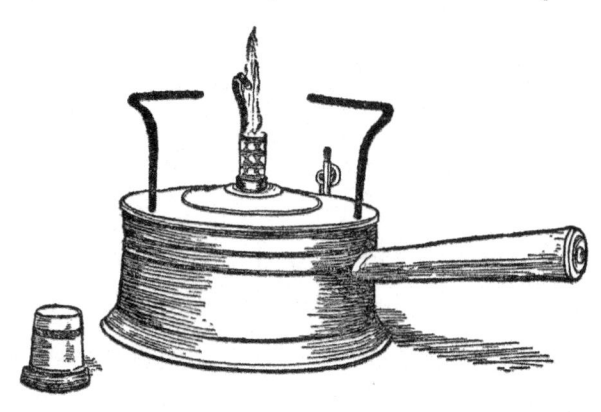

ALCOHOL IS SPLENDID TO BURN

If you put any dead animal, or a piece of flesh in alcohol, it will keep any length of time without spoiling. Doctors and scientists have all sorts of things carefully pickled in jars full of alcohol. In museums you can see many strange fishes, for instance, which look just as they did when first caught, although many years may have passed since they were put into those very jars.

Alcohol is used for many other useful things, especially in chemistry. Many of the pretty colors in which our clothes and ribbons are dyed could not have been made without alcohol. It is also used in mixing many kinds of medicines, and that is the main reason why you should never take any drugs save when the doctor tells you to do so.

Doctors know that alcohol can be used—just like arsenic and many other poisons—as *medicine* for certain diseases. They know all about the body and what it needs. They also know that there are times when the heart, for instance, beats too slowly, and when the extra beats which alcohol would cause, would do it good. At those times, when they are quite sure that the harm which alcohol does elsewhere cannot overbalance the good it may do to the heart, they order it for their patients.

When the doctor gives you some very horrid tasting medicine, you are never one bit anxious to take more doses than he tells you, and you often beg him to give you something else. But, when he gives you medicine which you learn to like, you not only fail to ask him to change it, but often go on taking it after he has told you it is not longer necessary to do so.

That is the great danger about alcohol when used as a medicine. People get to like it, and then they take more of it than the doctor wishes. Besides, when they find out that it *may* do good in certain cases of heart or stomach trouble, they often fancy it *must* do good in all, and, like the people of old, act as if they believed it a cure for all diseases.

A doctor who knows all about the human body, will give

alcohol (in some form) to one person, and none at all to the next, although the two may really have the same disease. He knows it will help one person to get well, but that it may make another very sick, and he alone can judge who should take it and how much they should take.

Alcohol is not the only medicine which is really harmful, that people like to take. Some learn to like opium, or morphine, or chloral, or some other drug, in which these poisons are mixed. Soon they cannot get along without it, take more and more, and finally they become very ill, or even crazy from the effects of these drugs.

It is because some of these poisons are so often found in patent medicines, that it is not at all safe to take them. There is poison in all the headache medicines and also in the soothing syrups. *Never,* never give your baby anything of the kind, for if you do not kill him outright, you may ruin his health, or his mind. In fact, the only safe rule is never to give or take any medicine that your doctor does not order, and to be sure and take only just as much of it as he tells you.

About Drinking

You have already been told that the only perfectly safe drinks are pure water, milk and slightly sweetened lemonade. There are, however, many others, which, if properly made, and if not taken too often, can do no great harm to any one. Cocoa and chocolate can feed as well as warm you, so they can be given even to little children, although there is a little poison in both.

Tea and coffee, freshly made, not too strong, and taken only at meal times, in reasonable quantities, do not hurt most *grown* people. But, like alcohol, tea and coffee are only cheats, for they make you think for a little while that you are stronger and livelier than you really are.

Besides, they are very apt to make children fidgety, to keep them awake when they should be asleep, to spoil their appetites more or less, to make them cross and disagreeable and to hinder their growth. So, children, leave tea and coffee entirely alone until you are twenty, and then it is not likely you will care to begin drinking them any more. I know some grown people who are very sorry because they have drunk coffee and tea all their lives, but I have never yet heard of any one who was sorry because he or she never drank either at all.

Your parents, who have taken tea and coffee ever since they were children, may think you foolish and cranky if you refuse to drink what they do, but you surely won't mind being teased a little, or even laughed at, if it is going to do you good and not harm in the end. If you must have something warm, drink hot water or hot milk.

Boys and girls, do practice self-denial and do not drink much soda water either. Remember that soda water is very bad for growing bones and teeth as well as for your stomach. Besides, by taking it, you get into the habit of drinking, and if you *must*

About Drinking

have soda when you are young, you will probably think you *must have* much stronger drinks when you are older. Those who "cannot resist" a glass of soda now, will not be able to "resist" taking a glass of some stronger drink later on.

If you teach yourself now to do without anything but milk and water, you will never regret it. About two thousand five hundred years ago a very wise man (Socrates) said: "Beware of those liquors which tempt you to drink when you are not thirsty, and of those foods which tempt you to eat when you are not hungry."

We have lived many hundreds of years since then, yet these words have never been found anything but true, and no one can give you wiser directions than those about what you should eat and drink.

The same wise man also said: "He who knows what is good and chooses it, who knows what is bad and avoids it, is learned and temperate." Now you can learn if you choose, what is good or bad for you, and any one who chooses the bad, after he knows that it is bad, fully deserves the punishment which is sure to overtake him sooner or later.

I would advise every girl who reads this book not only to be very careful about her own food and drink at all times, but when she grows up never to marry any man who is too self-indulgent in this matter. If she does, she may find herself with a drunken husband, sickly children, ruined health and leading a most unhappy life.

When it is thoroughly understood that no good woman will ever marry a man who drinks even a little, the men who expect to marry some day, and have homes and children of their own, will realize that they *must* keep away from temptation. So you see, girls, even if you cannot vote or change the laws, you can help to bring about a better state of things. Are you willing to do it?

QUESTIONS.—How was alcohol found, and what was it mistakenly called? What is the yeast plant; where is it found, and how does it act? Which are the best things for boys and girls to drink, and why? Do the Dwarfs like it when their master sends them any alcohol? Why does a man who drinks often want to go on drinking? For what reasons should you avoid the drink habit? Are people stronger with or without liquor? What stories show that liquor does not keep people warm? Do doctors feel sorry for people who suffer from the drink disease? How can you help a person who is trying to break the drink habit? Tell me some good ways to use alcohol? Are many drugs quite as bad as drink? Why should you refuse to drink tea and coffee until you are grown up, and why should you not have much soda water? Is it right for girls who know what you have read in this chapter to marry men who drink?

CHAPTER XIV

About Smoking and Chewing

UNTIL Christopher Columbus discovered America, and Sir Walter Raleigh brought the first tobacco to Europe, white men managed to live and be very happy without smoking at all. In fact, it was only about five hundred years ago that civilized men began to adopt what was probably one of the very worst of the savage customs, a custom which is doubly bad because it looks so very innocent.

At first, no one knew that tobacco—like drink—is only a cheat and a poison. Of course, tobacco always made men sick the first time they tried it, but as they believed it was quite harmless otherwise, they went on trying, until they learned to like it so well that they fancied they really could not get along without it.

The taste for tobacco, little by little, became so general that there are now more men who use it than men who do not, and so much money is spent every year for "the weed" as it is rightly called, that if that amount were set aside for a few years only, it is estimated we could pay off our immense national debt (in 1912, $2,831,330,305).

You see what huge sums of money go up in smoke every year, for even men whose families have to be supported by charity always have money to burn in this way.

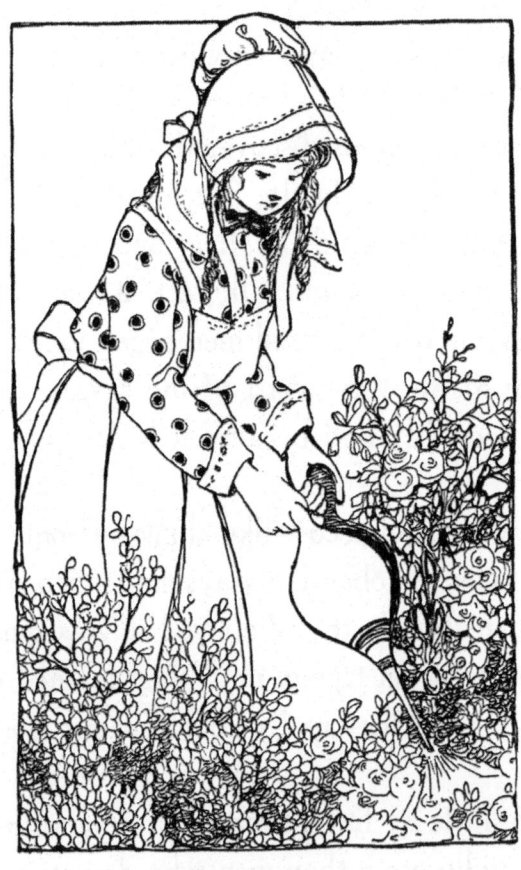

Even doctors who smoke themselves, will tell you that tobacco is a poison, that it is bad for the teeth, bad for the throat, bad for the lungs, bad for the stomach, bad for the heart, bad for the skin, and bad for the brain. Besides, they will tell you that, unlike alcohol, tobacco has no good side at all, save that it is useful in gardens and greenhouses to kill bugs and other vermin.

TOBACCO IS USEFUL IN GARDENS—TO KILL BUGS

Of course, men who only smoke a little, and who use tobacco which is clean and not too strong, do not suffer enough from its bad effects to notice them greatly.

But even when they do, they *like* tobacco so much, that they are not willing to admit that it can have any share in making them ill, or to give up using it.

Many doctors got into the habit of smoking before they knew of all the harm that tobacco can do. Others began using it when they were medical students, simply because they had to work many hours a day over things which smelled so very bad that it was a great relief to have a strong odor always under their noses to deaden the rest.

These doctors will tell you that by the time they were through their disagreeable work, the *habit* of smoking had become so deeply rooted, that they no longer *wished* to give it up. Still, they cannot but add, that they and every one else would be much better off, if they never smoked at all. They also say that it is estimated that a young man who learns to smoke or chew, wilfully destroys one fifth of the enjoyment and value of his life and one tenth of its length.

Although men can become insane as the result of too much smoking or chewing, tobacco does not have such plainly seen bad effects as alcohol, so it is never considered half as bad to smoke as to drink. In fact, any number of very good men use tobacco every day. But they certainly would never have gotten into the habit of doing so, if they had learned in time what harm it could work them and others, for really *good* men are never wilfully selfish.

After a man—even a very good one—has once learned to

smoke or chew, it becomes an almost hopeless task to convince him that he is doing wrong, or make him give it up. You see, there are too many brain cells stowed away in his self-indulgent storehouse, all full of excuses for doing as he wishes.

This book is not written with any hope of changing grown-ups, whose habits are already fixed. It is merely intended to save you boys and girls from *forming* bad habits, and to show you plainly how foolish it is to ruin one's own life for the sake of pleasing a taste which you have not yet learned, and which you would have to cultivate.

If you see grown up persons who *want* to give up drinking or smoking, help and encourage them as much as you can, but do not bother them or preach to them. Your business is to look after yourselves and your own companions. *You* are warned against the bad habits which you might adopt, and if, after that, *you* go ahead and form them, you will be much more blameworthy than the older people, whom perhaps you now secretly despise for being so self-indulgent and so foolish, to say the least.

The Harm Tobacco Can Do

We have said that no one can deny that much tobacco must harm the person who uses it and that most moderate smokers, when asked to give their honest opinion, will confess that it is much wiser not to smoke or chew at all.

Men declare that they smoke because it soothes them, because it rests them, because it helps their digestion, because it makes them think better or quicker, because they are lonely and because it keeps them company, because they have nothing else to do, and because others smoke, and it is more sociable to do as others do.

All these reasons, to a person who has stored no "tobacco cells" away in his brain, seem very childish and foolish and really good for nothing. Some doctors who liked to smoke, and wished therefore to prove that there is some truth in these reasons, have been obliged to own up frankly that they cannot do so. They even say that a great deal of their practice is due to the harm which tobacco does to the body.

As our bodies were given us in trust, we have no right to harm them in any way. We have no right either to injure our minds or our characters, and still it is pretty generally agreed that the use of tobacco does both. A good man who smokes and chews, would be a far better man if he did neither, and you have surely never yet heard of any one so good that he or she could afford not to try to be a little better.

Besides a man who smokes or chews cannot give his children as strong nerves as if he did neither, and every man ought to think of his children's welfare.

General Grant and Emperor Frederick of Germany, who were both great and good men, nevertheless smoked so much that it gave them cancer of the throat from which they died. It is also said that President McKinley might perhaps have recovered from his wound if he had not had a "smoker's heart," for smoking wears the heart out by making it beat faster than it should.

Now, Grant, McKinley and Frederick were unusually strong men, and if tobacco can do so much harm to *strong* men, you can imagine what havoc it plays with those who are not strong. A doctor counted the heart-beats of a smoker, and found that after eleven minutes' smoking, it beat thirty-eight beats a minute more! Doctors also tell us that tobacco makes many men crazy or that it brings about attacks of paralysis.

It is said that the most moderate smoker spends forty dollars a year for tobacco. Now, if these forty dollars were laid aside every year, from the time he was twenty until he was sixty, this man could buy a nice little home to live in during his old age.

A man who kept exact accounts, died in Vienna recently. He had smoked 628,713 cigars in forty-six years. You can count for yourselves how much money this man burned, even if he smoked the very cheapest kind of cigars—those made in a dirty way from cigar ends picked up in the gutter!

How Tobacco Acts on Boys

It has been proved that bad as tobacco is for men, it is much worse for boys who have not yet reached their full growth. It dwarfs and stunts them body and mind, and injures their characters as well.

A doctor once examined thirty-eight boys under fifteen who were known to smoke. He found that although these boys had been quite healthy before they began to use tobacco, twenty-seven of them had already gotten diseases which no doctor could ever entirely cure. Some of them had the seeds of diseases which would make them unhappy and useless all their lives.

The remaining eleven boys were stupid and lazy, and complained of headache and sore eyes, although they were not yet really sick. Still, some of them felt even worse than the boys who had diseases which would soon send them to their graves.

Now, just think whether it paid to smoke! Here were thirty-eight boys who could have been good men and useful citizens, but they threw away all their chances for the sake of pleasing their vanity and their taste for tobacco.

It is so well proved that tobacco is bad for the health, that no athlete is ever allowed to use it, in any form, while in training. Besides, in Switzerland there are laws forbidding the sale of tobacco to boys under fifteen, and if one is caught using the weed he is arrested and punished.

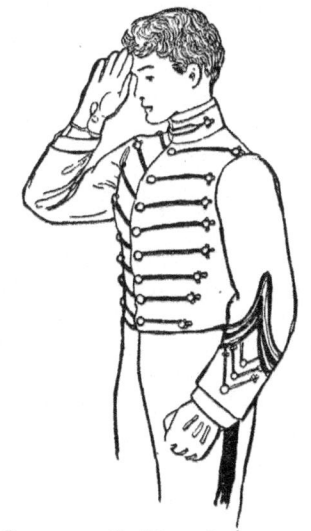

SMOKING IS NOT ALLOWED AT WEST POINT

In Germany—the land of smokers—the law forbids the use

of tobacco to all youths under sixteen. Smoking is not allowed at West Point, at Annapolis or in the State Military School in Paris, for the American and French governments have found out that a student who smokes is not nearly as bright as when he does not smoke, and that he is not likely to do so well in his profession.

While only some of the good men smoke, all the bad ones do, so Horace Greeley used to say: "Show me a genuine blackguard who is not fond of tobacco in some way, and I will show you two white blackbirds!"

Every year, ten pounds of chewing tobacco, three and a half pounds of smoking, and a half pound of snuff are made in the United States for every male person, and six hundred million cigarettes are sold to supply the wants of six million youths! All this tobacco has to be grown, manufactured and sold, so many people are employed. But if the people thus employed had known the harm that tobacco can do, I feel very sure that few of them would care to have anything to do with it. They would surely rather grow, manufacture and sell something else.

Because liquor and tobacco *can* do harm, the people who make and sell these things, are often looked down upon by others. We now know that those who are doing it may be excusable, but if their children do not see other and better ways of making money, when old enough to choose for themselves, they will deserve all the contempt which they are likely to meet some years hence, when everybody will have become fully aware of the ruin which tobacco as well as drink can bring about.

GIRLS AND TOBACCO

If all the girls in our country banded together and refused to have anything to do with the boys who smoked, they would soon bring about a great change. They would, in the same time, benefit themselves greatly, for later on, when they grow up and want to marry, they will be very glad indeed to have husbands who do not selfishly burn money which might do good to their family or to the poor. Besides, their own health will be far better if they don't have to breathe air spoiled by tobacco smoke. Their children will be stronger and less likely to die in babyhood, and all their home life will be purer and happier.

Girls, is not that worth trying for, even now? You will be teased and laughed at, but you are surely brave enough to stand a little of that. Just give the boys to understand, once for all, that while you are not such little prigs as to find fault with anything your fathers or uncles may choose to do, you are going to have your say about what your companions do, and that you certainly never mean to marry a man too weak-minded and self-indulgent to do what is proved to be right and to avoid forming bad habits.

A girl, even in fun, or out of daring, should never touch a cigar or cigarette. You may be told that *fine* ladies do it, but *nice* ladies do not. Noble women shrink from the mere thought of such a thing. A woman who knows what harm smoking can do to the health, and who nevertheless smokes, is a woman of no character or principle.

As much as you can keep out of smoky air, for every whiff of it is bad for your health. Girls brought up in homes where the air is blue with smoke, can never be quite as healthful and strong as they would have been had the air they breathed night and day always been quite pure. They are also more likely to have sickly children who will feel the bad effects from it, as I will explain to you later on.

That every inch of a tobacco user's body is tainted by the poison, is proved by the fact that cannibals,—who like to eat what they call "long pig"—refuse to touch the flesh of any person who has smoked a great deal. If we lived among cannibals, it *might* pay to smoke so as not to be eaten, but as it is, there is really no excuse whatever for a new generation growing up to make the same awful mistake as their fathers and grandfathers.

About Chewing

A man or boy who chews tobacco, suffers often even more from its evil effects than a smoker. Do you want to know why? It is because a smoker draws in only a little of the poison from his pipe, cigar or cigarette, and blows out the rest to poison others, while a chewer swallows a great deal of it without meaning to do so.

If he swallowed all the spittle flavored with tobacco, which

About Chewing

he has in his mouth all the time, it would soon make him very ill and even kill him. To avoid being sick at his stomach, a tobacco chewer spits all the time. This is a filthy, disgusting habit, and as I have already explained to you the danger to others of spitting in anything but your handkerchief, or spittoon, you can understand why almost everybody now objects to that mode of using tobacco. Still, while little disease germs may rise from the dried spittle and do much mischief, a man who chews tobacco does not spoil all the air around him as a smoker does, and is hence less offensive to many people.

Some school children are very fond of chewing-gum. They like it because it is nicely flavored with peppermint or vanilla, and because as long as they keep it in their mouths, that good taste tickles their palate. If the chewing-gum is well made, there is no poison whatever in it, so you might therefore think that it can do no harm at all to those who chew it.

But you are greatly mistaken. Chewing-gum is really very bad for everybody. You remember, do you not, what I told you about the spittle buckets in your little house? Well, as long as your jaws move, and as long as there is something in your mouth, those spittle buckets work hard to moisten it.

All this spittle is swallowed again and again and the little buckets get no rest at all. They work and work. All the spittle they make is wasted, because it was meant to digest food, and chewing-gum is not food but a cheat.

The spittle buckets get so tired and use up so much good material wetting that stupid stuff, that when meal time comes, and you eat good food, they cannot supply really good spittle enough to digest it. Then the food goes down into the stomach only partly moistened and sweetened, and the poor Stomach Dwarf gets very cross because he has too much extra work to do.

He says for instance: "Here I have been trotting to the stairway, every few minutes all day, because telegrams came that something had been swallowed and that I must see to it! Each time I looked, I found a swallow of spittle, flavored with wintergreen or some other stuff like that! The very idea of wasting spittle and of disturbing me for nothing. I think master must have taken leave of his senses! If he doesn't look out I'll get mad, for while I am ready to work, I hate to be fooled!"

Children who must chew something all the time—a piece of paper, or a bit of rubber when they cannot get anything else—are doing great harm to their spittle buckets as you see. When they grow up, chewing will be such a habit, that they will feel unhappy and lost without something in their mouths, and then they may take to chewing tobacco!

Many mothers—who do not know what harm they are doing—give their babies rubber nipples to suck whenever they whimper or cry. The babies,—whose instinct is to suck whatever is put into their mouths—then stop crying, for they cannot suck and cry at the same time. This is all mothers want. But they do not know that all the time a baby sucks that rubber, his poor little spittle buckets have to work very hard.

When real food is given him after awhile, the tired spittle buckets cannot make good spittle, the food does not digest well, the baby frets more and more, and every one wonders why that child has such a weak stomach!

Never let your baby begin to suck a rubber nipple or his thumb. Stop it every time he tries it, and he'll soon get into good habits. It may give you a little more trouble at first, but it is sure to give you less in the end, and it is far, far better for the darling's health.

QUESTIONS.—Who discovered America, and who brought tobacco from America to Europe? Did people know at first that there was any harm in the innocent-looking tobacco plant? Do most men use tobacco, and why? Should you preach to older people who smoke? Whom should you watch over and teach good habits? Is tobacco particularly bad for growing boys, and why? Are athletes who are training for a match or race allowed to use tobacco? Do you want to store tobacco-cells in your brain? Could the money spent for tobacco be put to a better use? Should girls refuse to associate with boys who smoke? Is it wise or nice for girls to smoke? Why is chewing-gum bad for your health, and how does the Stomach Dwarf like it? Why should not a baby suck its thumb or a rubber nipple? How can you give the baby good habits?

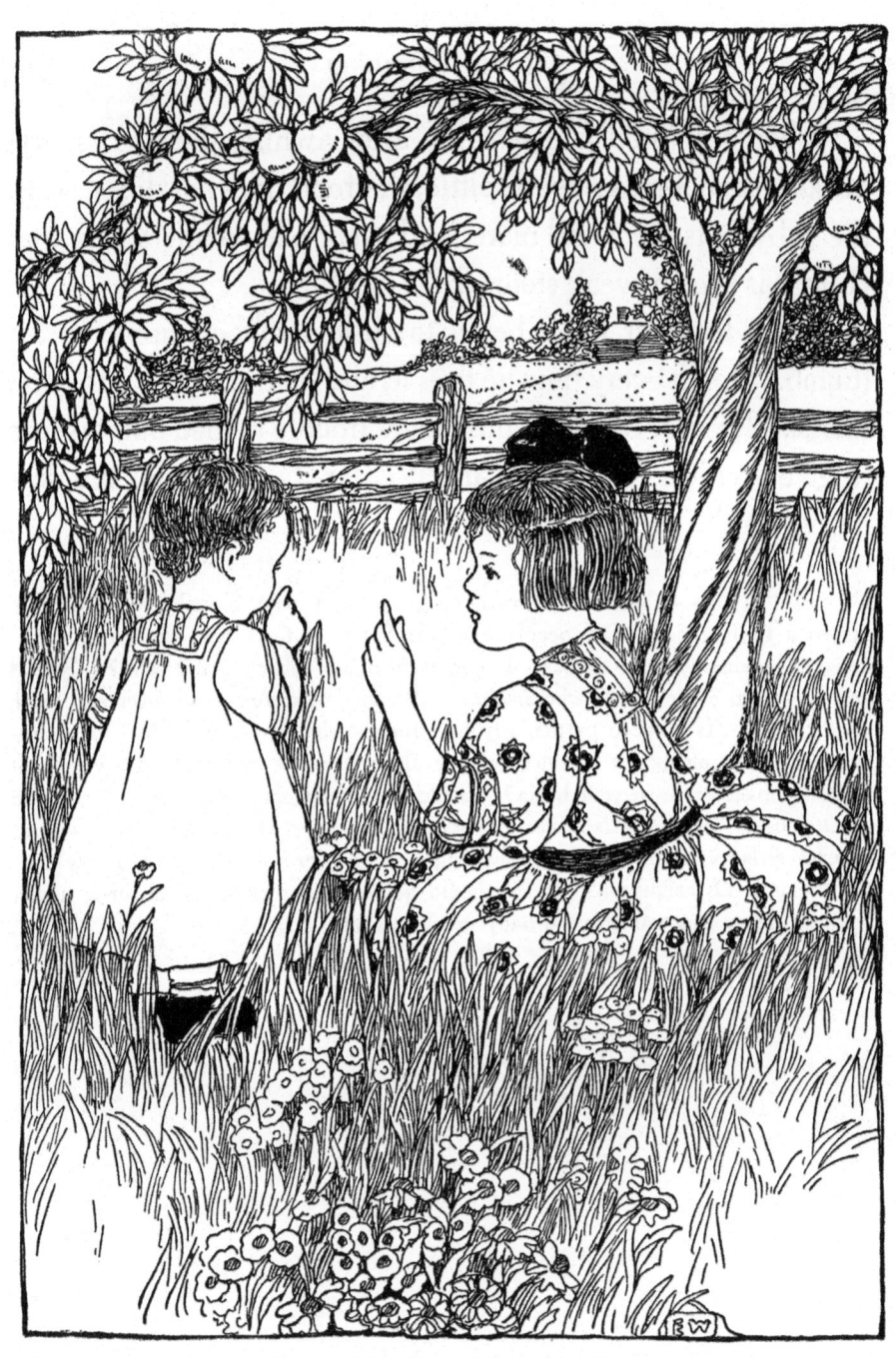

DON'T LET BABY SUCK HIS THUMB

CHAPTER XV

PLANT, FISH, BIRD AND ANIMAL BABIES

DID you ever go to your father or mother for help in your arithmetic, for instance, and find out that while they could *do* your sums and get the right answers, they often did them in a very different way from your teacher, and could not explain to you as clearly the reasons why they did them so?

Father and mother—especially if they are older—may know even more than your teacher does, but as it is not their business to teach arithmetic, they do not know the best and shortest way to go to work about it. Each person, you know, has his or her own trade or work, and while your mother may be the best mother, or housekeeper, or dressmaker, or artist there ever was, she may not be a good teacher.

Your father may be the best plumber, doctor, waiter, musician, or bookkeeper in the whole country, and still not be able to *teach* arithmetic.

Of course a few parents have a gift for teaching and explaining, and thus can do it better than any one else; but many others know so well that they cannot teach, that they are very glad to have you go to school and learn from others all you need know.

It is because most parents don't know how to explain hard things in an easy way, that they so often say: "Oh, don't bother me!" "Ask some one else," or "You couldn't understand even if I were to tell you," or "You must wait until you grow up before you can understand that!"

Some parents also think that as they cannot explain many true things in such a way that their children will understand, they must satisfy them by telling them fairy-tales or nonsense. As you know, there is some very pleasant nonsense which makes you laugh, and there is provoking nonsense which makes you angry. The loveliest of all fairy-tales, and the very nicest nonsense there ever was, is the story of Santa Claus.

Now that you are no longer babies, you probably know or guess that Santa Claus never lived at all, and that the reindeers, the visit down each chimney, the sleighful of toys, and all the rest, is just make-believe of the very nicest kind. Your parents enjoyed it all so much when they were little, that they wanted you to have the same fun too, while you could, and therefore they let you believe what was not true.

Christmas is never half so merry when one no longer believes in Santa Claus, so they let you read and talk about him all you pleased, and never told you that it was all a fairy-tale until they had to.

Besides, Christmas—the birthday of Christ—means so much that is beautiful and holy to most Christian parents, that they always think it better to wait until children are old enough to understand, before they tell them all the story of the Child born in a manger, whose birth proved such a blessing to all the world, although His life was so sad.

The longer you live and the older you get, the clearer you will see that it is always hardest to talk of the things we care about most. For instance, you can easily tell me how much you love your cat, your bicycle, your doll or your ball, but when you want to tell your mother how dearly you love her,

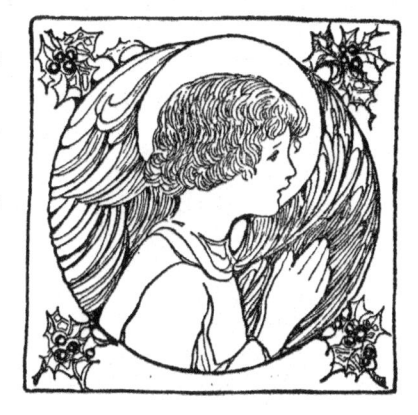

CHRISTMAS IS BEAUTIFUL AND HOLY

you can only hug and kiss her and say, over and over again: "I love you, ever and ever so much!"

Many good fathers and mothers feel so deeply about religion, that they seldom talk about it, but expect their children to learn all about it in church, in Sunday-school, and from their books. In the same way, many fathers and mothers—who know all about being parents and where all the babies come from—often cannot answer your simplest question about that, because they feel it too deeply.

Some of them feel so very deeply that they say: "Oh, don't tell the children anything about it! They cannot understand yet. Just let them believe any fairy-tale they please, but don't tell them the truth. Let them find out all about it only by and by, when they are much older."

But I am sure you are already quite old enough to understand, provided it is made clear to you. I am therefore going to tell you truly how all the babies—the plant babies, the fish babies, the bird babies, the animal babies, and the human babies—come into the world. This is what is often called "Nature's Secret."

Now you surely all know that secrets are very sacred, and very precious. We tell secrets only to persons whom we know we can trust, and it is because I feel sure I can trust you, that I am telling you now. Remember that you must *keep* any secret which is trusted to you. That is to say you must not talk about it to any one, unless the person who told it to you says you may.

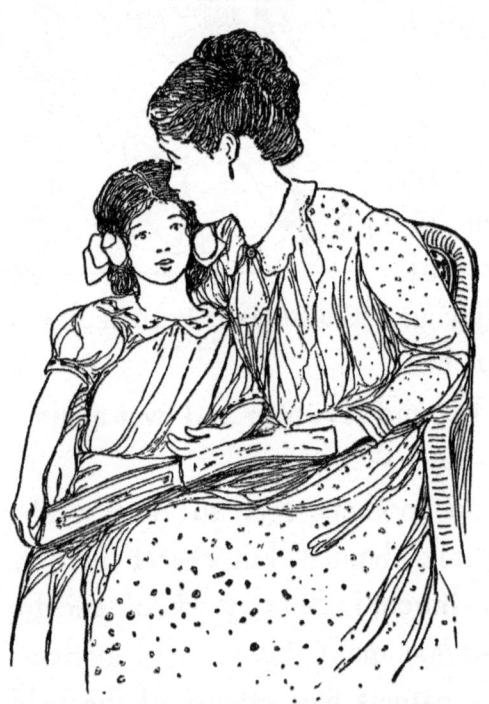

A Secret Between Mother and You

You may talk to mother about "Nature's Secret," as much as you please, and you may talk about it to your teacher if you read this book in school, but all the rest of the time I expect you not to say one word about it to any one else, and to keep it to yourself. Children who are true, and who have a nice sense of honor, can always be trusted, and I feel sure, though I cannot look straight into your eyes that *you* can be trusted. So show yourselves worthy of this trust by not talking at all about sacred matters like this to any one except your mother.

All the grown up people know all about Nature's secret, so you see it is really no secret at all, but it is *called* a secret because it is a very sacred and private matter, which nice-minded people never mention lightly.

ABOUT PLANT BABIES

You have already heard that plants are alive, that they eat and drink, as it were, that they breathe and that they grow. When God made the first tree, the first plant, and the first blade of grass or bit of moss, He made it as a pattern. He did not wish to go on forever and ever making all the trees, plants, grass and moss, needed to cover the bare earth with beauty, and to give food to animals and man, so He gave each living thing the power to make others just like itself.

Every plant, tree, blade of grass, and every bit of moss, was to grow, bloom, and bear fruit or seed, and from this seed, new plants, new trees, new blades of grass, and new bits of moss were to grow, just like the pattern first made by God.

You may not know that God also decided that all living things should be one of two kinds, or sexes, that is to say, either male or female. There are therefore male and female plants, male and female fishes, male and female birds and other animals, and men and women, or male and female human beings.

God wanted creatures of the same kind to love each other, and be kind to one another, so He also divided all living things into families. There are plant families, as well as animal and human families, and when you come to study in higher classes, you will learn much more than I can tell you here about the plant, animal and human families.

There are plant families, as we have said. These families have different ways of living and of bringing up their children. Sometimes the father and mother live on the same plant, and even in the same flower-house. Sometimes the father lives in one flower-house and the mother in another.

When f a t h e r and mother live in the same flower-house, they can settle their family affairs all alone, but when they live on different plants, or in different flower-houses, they have to send messages to one another by the bees, the butterflies and the wind.

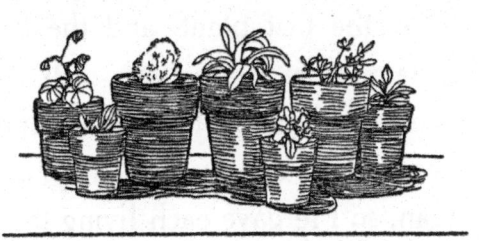

PLANT BABIES

To make you understand just what takes place, I am going to make believe that the flowers talk. They *may* talk really, but as it is not any language we can hear or understand, we often say that they cannot speak.

Whenever the flowers open wide, you can see, down in the centre of each father flower, some pretty yellow dust. When this yellow dust is ready to drop or fly away, the father flower says: "Here is some nice yellow dust. God has hidden away in each little speck of this yellow dust the power to grow into a plant just like me. But this dust is so small and so delicate, that it can easily get lost. I wish I knew of some nice safe place where I could hide it, where it would be warm, could get food, and grow nicely."

Then the mother flower calls out: "Hidden away here, down by my heart, there is a dear little nest, which God bade me make as a cradle for flower babies. Just send me your yellow dust. I'll tuck it away here safely, and take good care of it. We'll see if it can really grow up into a flower baby, although it is so very small now."

Then the father plant either shakes his yellow dust down upon the mother plant, or the wind, or the bees, or the butterflies carry it over to her.

The tiny specks of yellow dust slip down a little passage, or tube, which leads right to the little flower nest, where they are safely tucked away by the mother plant. There, the mother brings them food and air, and there they grow and grow bigger and bigger.

If the flower cradle did not grow bigger and bigger too, the flower babies would soon be much too large for their nests. The flower mother is so busy seeing that her babies have food and air enough (it is all carried to them by the sap-boats, just as food is carried to our muscles by the blood-boats), that she quite forgets to look after herself at all.

Her pretty dress fades and grows ragged, her bright color fades away, and one fine day, the weary flower-mother says: "My work is all done! My flower babies are fine and strong. I am so tired, I think now that they don't need me any more at all, I'll just go to sleep!"

Then the tired flower-mother goes to sleep, never to wake up again, for her work in the world is all done; and whenever there is nothing more God wishes a flower, an animal or a human being to do, He takes back the life which He gave them.

The flower babies don't get any more food now, but they feel big and restless. Their nest seems much too small. They stretch and stretch, until one fine day the thin walls of their little room or nest crack, and all the flower babies, or seeds tumble out and fall on the ground.

Some of these flower babies—for there are often ever so many of them tucked away in the same little room—are eaten up by the birds, some dried up by the sun, some soaked and spoiled by the rain, but a few get trodden into the ground, where they lie safely, until they begin to sprout and grow there in their own way.

Get a pea, or a bean, or a morning-glory seed,—any seed is a plant baby, you know,—plant it and see it grow. The seed swells, the shell or skin cracks, a tiny root pushes downward, little leaves push upward, and before long you have a plant, just like the father and mother of that baby seed.

Even big oak-trees grow up out of tiny acorns, and oaks, as well as bits of grass, once had a father and a mother. In time, when baby plants grow big enough, they will be either father or mother to other trees or plants just like themselves. Now you know exactly where all the plant babies come from, for I have told you the whole truth in this easy way.

THE FISH BABIES

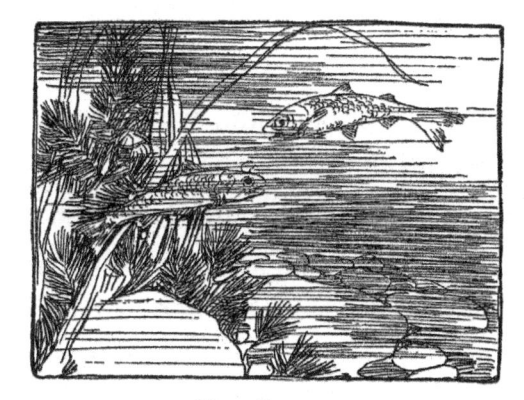

FISH BABIES

Fishes live in the water. As water is cold and chills warm-blooded creatures, all fishes have cold blood, or at least blood not nearly so warm as ours. It is always said that cold-blooded creatures are far less loving than those with warm blood, so you will not be surprised to hear that most fishes do not care very much for their little babies.

There are male and female, or father and mother fishes, just as there are male and female plants. It was God who made the first fishes, and gave them the power to make other fishes like themselves.

You often have fish for dinner, do you not? Well, once in a while, mother gets what is known as a roe-fish. You know, do you not, that before chickens or fishes are cooked, they are always opened. The insides are carefully taken out and thrown away, before the chicken or fish is cooked.

When mother buys a roe-fish, you find in its belly, besides the parts you throw away, many, many tiny little round things, which look like beads, and which are all wrapped up in a fine but very strong skin, which keeps them apart from the bowels and all the rest of the fish.

These bead-like things are fish eggs, and they are never found except at certain times, in the body of a female fish.

God made in the body of the first female fish, a little skin room, in which many, many eggs could grow. In spring, when the water gets nice and warm, these tiny eggs—they are made and fed by the fish blood-boats which bring them air and food,—swell and swell, and when they reach the right size, the female fish begins to look around for a nice place where she can hide them.

Most fishes like to lay their eggs in some river or brook, where they think baby-fishes can thrive best, so the mother fishes swim away to find the mouths of rivers or brooks.

As there are male as well as female fishes, the females soon meet male fishes, swimming around in the lakes or seas. Now, as I want you to know just what happens, we'll make believe that fishes talk.

The Fish Babies

The male fish says: "When God made the first male fish, He gave him the power to give life to other fishes just like himself. In my body there is a liquid. If I could only pour it over some fish eggs, I am sure there would soon be nice little fishes just like me. I wonder where I can find some fish eggs?"

Then the female fish says: "I know. If you come with me, I will show you. I have some nice fish eggs. You can be father, and I'll be mother to a big family of fish babies!" Then the two fishes swim off together.

By and by they come to a place where the water is nice and still, where the sand is fine, where the sun shines warmly, and the mother-fish says: "Here is a nice place. I am going to lay the eggs, which are hidden away in a little nest in my body, right here!"

Then the door to the little egg room opens, and the eggs drop out on the fine sand. When the mother fish has laid all her eggs, the father fish comes swimming along, and when he sees those nice eggs he pours out over them the liquid which is in his body. Then all the eggs which are touched by the liquid can grow and grow, until they become baby-fishes. But those which the father liquid does not touch never grow at all, they spoil and are lost.

Some father and mother fishes stay around near their eggs, to watch them until the tiny baby fishes break out of the fish eggs, begin to swim around, and can look after themselves. But other father and mother fishes swim away just as soon as their egg-nest is made. You see, they are cold-blooded, and so do not have much affection for their young.

As there are hundreds and thousands of fish eggs in the body of one female fish, you can easily imagine how many baby fishes there are. But, as many big fishes feed on small ones, ever and ever so many of these baby fishes are eaten up, long before they can grow up to be father and mother fishes in their turn. Were it not so, there would soon be so many fishes in the sea, that they would be packed there as tightly as they are now in the boxes of salt fish, which we buy at the grocer's!

Some of you children who live in the country, may have seen in spring, in a frog-pond, what looked like a big lump of whitish gelatine with many little black specks all through it. These black specks are the eggs laid by mother frog, and in time they will hatch into polliwogs or baby frogs. Although father frog—like all fishes—is said to be cold-blooded, the life fluid he poured over the eggs was so much warmer than the water, that it jellied, just as any hot syrup does if you drop it in cold water. That is why the black specks are all covered with transparent white jelly.

Now, you know exactly how the baby-fishes and baby frogs come into the world, do you not?

The Bird Babies

Birds can move even quicker than fishes. They live mostly in the air, flying about. As it takes a great deal more strength

The Bird Babies

to fly in the air than to swim in the water, the blood of the birds flows around much quicker than the blood of the fishes. Because it flows so much quicker, it is warmer, in fact, birds are the warmest blooded of all creatures.

Now I told you that the warmer the blood the better the mind, and the more affection the parents showed to their young. So you will not be surprised to hear that father and mother birds look after their young much better than father and mother fish.

There are male and female birds of every kind. God, in the beginning, gave all the birds He made, power to make or create other birds like themselves, that is to say, to pass on the life which He had given them to their young, so that even when they were all dead and gone, there would still be other birds to fly around, and delight us by their beauty and song, and to teach us lessons of patience and love.

Early in the spring, when the baby birds of last summer are full grown male and female birds, they begin to feel that they ought to do something more than eat and drink, fly about and sing, and that they should use the power which God gave them and pass on some of their joyous life to other birds. So the young male birds begin to sing. As I want you to know what it is they sing, I'll put the song you have so often heard, into words which you can understand, just as well as any of the female birds who hear it.

The male bird sings: "Here! Here! look at me! As fine a bird as ever you'd see! I can fly, I can sing, I am young, I am strong. Last summer my brothers, my sisters and I were all bird babies up in a dear little nest in a shady tree. I remember that nest well. I remember how father and mother flew around all day long, getting such nice fat worms and flies and slugs for us to eat!

"I'd like to build a nest just like that one, up in the fork of some nice tree. But I'd like to have some one to help me, just as my mother helped my father. Isn't there any nice little female bird who'd be willing to help me? We could build that nest together. We could line it with nice soft moss and feathers. Then she could lay some pretty eggs in it. While she hatched those eggs, I would sit up on a branch and sing to her. I'd go and get nice worms to feed to her. Whenever she wanted to stretch her legs or wings I'd sit on those dear little eggs so as to keep them nice and warm until she came back. Then, when the baby birds came out of the shells, I'd help her feed them, I'd hunt worms and slugs all day long.

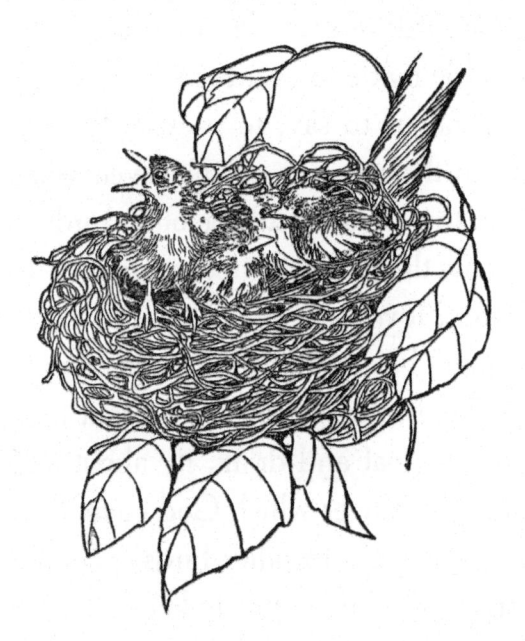

BIRD BABIES

"When evening came, and she tucked our babies safe under her wing, I'd sing a little song to put them to sleep, before I put my own weary head under my wing to go to sleep too. I'd wake up first in the morning, when the very first pink or yellow glow appeared in the east, and as soon as I heard my little wife's first chirp, I'd pour out a glad morning song before we started out together to take our morning bath and get the wee babies' breakfast.

"When our babies got big enough to fly, she and I would teach them how to look after themselves, and when they grew so big and strong that they did not need us any longer, my little wife and I would fly away together to the sunny South, where we would spend the long, cold winter."

More About Bird Babies

You heard in our last chapter what the male bird sings. By and by, a female bird, who has no mate as yet, but who is looking around for some one to help *her* build a nest, listens to his song. She says: "Are you quite sure, you big, strong bird, that you won't get tired waiting on me during the long weeks I'll have to sit on my eggs, so as to keep them warm and hatch out baby birds? If you are selfish, if you want to fly off to have a good time, I'll starve, or else I'll have to leave my eggs uncovered. Eggs can soon grow cold, you know, and a mere chill would be quite enough to kill my babies. Then, too, even after they come safely out of the shell, you and I will have to work very hard, or our babies will starve. Are you quite sure you can be a good and patient husband and father? Are you quite sure you can forget your own comfort to think only of me and of our babies for a while?"

If the male bird can satisfy the female bird, so that she feels she can trust him, they mate, that is to say, they become bird husband and wife, and go off together to build their nest. The female bird soon finds out that the male bird is always ready to give her the nicest worms he finds, to carry the heaviest sticks and the longest straws, and that he is cheerful and good tempered, and ready to sing to her when she wakes up and when she goes to sleep.

Bird husband and wife learn to love each other dearly, and if you watch pigeons, for instance, you will see and hear them billing and cooing, which is bird way of kissing each other and calling each other pet names.

Mated birds are husband and wife, so of course they are very intimate and tell each other all their secrets, and things no one else need know. As birds' eggs have hard shells, and the life fluid cannot soak through those, the father bird gives some of his to the mother bird, who stows it away in the eggs before the hard shell grows all around them.

Three, four, five or more eggs are always laid in each nest, and the hard shell around them prevents their being crushed flat, when the mother bird begins to sit upon them so as to hatch them. In each little egg, there is a tiny speck or drop of life-fluid, so that it can change and grow into a baby bird, or young chick, if kept warm enough. In each egg there is also stowed away all the food each little bird will need until he is strong enough to break his shell. This food is what is called the white and yolk of the egg. And up at one end, you can also find a little supply of air for the baby bird to breathe.

For about three weeks, the mother bird—who never kept still for a moment in her life before except when she was asleep, —sits on these eggs with outspread wings, to keep them snug and warm. She sits quite still, although it is keen torture for her, and while she sits there so patiently, the father bird gets her nice worms to eat, sings pretty songs to cheer her, and helps and encourages her all he can.

When she has to leave the nest for a few minutes every day, to stretch her poor cramped legs, and flutter her stiff wings, the father bird sits upon the eggs to keep them warm. But he soon grows weary of this work, and is very glad indeed when the mother bird comes back again. You see, each one has special duties, and as the father bird's work is to rush around and get food, of course he would rather do that.

One fine day, the mother bird calls to the father bird: "Oh, my dear, my dear! I do believe our bird babies are soon going to creep out of their shells. I hear a faint noise. It sounds like 'pick! pick!' just as if they were tapping their little bills against the shells to peck their way out!"

Father and mother bird are very much excited, and sure

enough, before long baby birds come creeping out of their shells, to receive a loving welcome. The empty, broken shells are quickly flung out of the nest, and as the new bird babies shiver with cold, the mother bird covers them close with her soft feathers, until they feel quite warm, and dry, and happy.

After awhile the baby birds begin to say: "Peep! peep!" which means: "I am hungry! I am so hungry! give me something to eat!"

The father and mother bird are kept very busy during the next few weeks feeding these hungry babies. At first, they chew all the food for them, and give it to them only when it is nice and soft; but after a while, the bird babies are able to eat whole worms and grain, nice fat slugs, and bits of ripe cherries and berries. Then they grow big and soon tumble out of the nest and learn to fly.

Your father and mother often say they have their hands pretty full looking after the wants of one baby at a time, but father and mother bird always have several babies at once to bring up, so you can imagine how very busy and tired they must be.

It is because birds are such very good parents, because they are so loving, so tender, so patient and so active, that they are often held up to us as examples, and all those who love and understand birds, can learn a great deal of good from them.

You have now heard how all the bird babies come into the

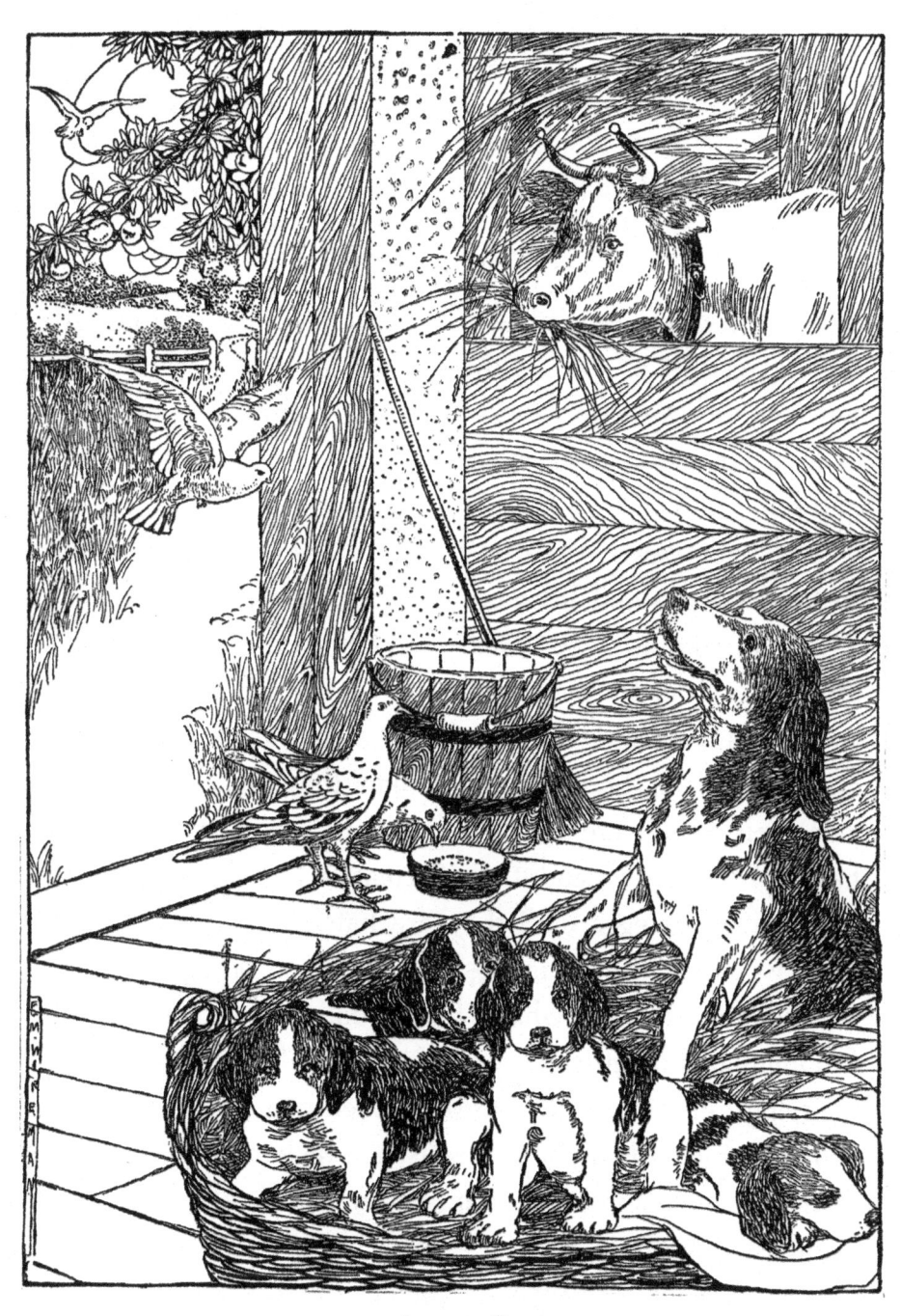

Animal Babies

world, and I hope you have also learned a little how beautiful the life of a bird family can be.

Animal Babies

As you have seen, plant babies and fish babies look after themselves just as soon as they break out of the seed, or egg, in which they are safely tucked away. There are so very many of them, that it does not matter if some are lost, some starved, and some eaten up. There are still plenty left.

Bird babies are not nearly so plentiful as fish or plant babies, so they are guarded far more carefully while they are young and small, and allowed to leave the home nest only when quite able to look out for themselves.

Besides birds and fishes, there are, as you know, many, many other animals in the world. The finer they are, the more delicate their babies are apt to be, and the more carefully they have to be nursed when little. A creature as light as a bird, can easily sit upon eggs until they are hatched, but just imagine what would happen if an elephant had to sit on eggs!

God always knows what is best to do, so when He made the first animals, He settled that ever so many of them should hatch their eggs, inside and not outside of their own bodies. All the animals which do this, have breasts, in which milk comes to feed their young when they are born, so they are all called mammals, or breast animals.

There are male and female animals of each kind among the

mammals, to whom God has given the power to make other animal bodies just like themselves. Just as every plant, and fish and bird, has to have a father and mother, all the mammals have to have fathers and mothers too.

You all know that cows give milk, so cows are mammals, are they not? In the cow's body, as in the bird's and the fish's, there is a little room, which God provided as a home for the cow's baby. Here the cow blood-boats bring air, and food, and material to make a tiny egg. This egg is very, very small and soft, although the cow is so very big, but when the life fluid once gets into it, it begins to grow. In a little while it hatches into a baby calf. The calf stays in the little room, where the cow blood-boats bring it all the air and food it needs, and plenty of material so that it can grow.

When it is big and strong, the door opens, and the calf drops out, or is born, as we often call it. The mother cow then licks her calf to show it how dearly she loves it, and when the calf stands up on

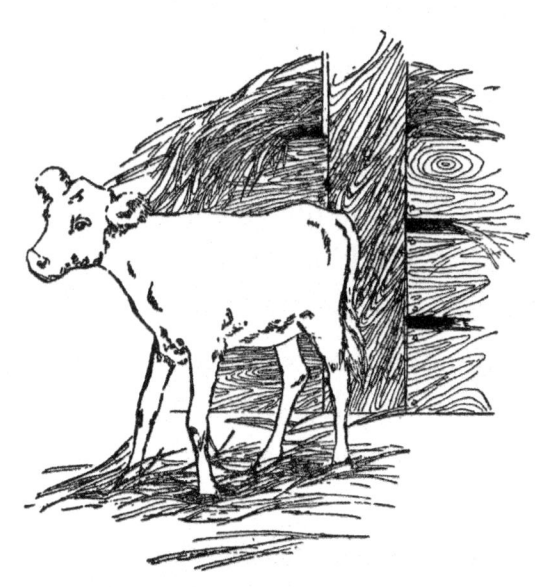

A SHAKY-LEGGED CALF

its long, shaky legs, and says in calf-talk: "I am hungry!" the mother answers:

"Well, my dear, God knew you would be hungry, so He sent some milk into my milk bag (the cow's breast). Just help yourself, my dear, suck all you want." If you have ever seen baby calves feed, you will know that they are very greedy little things, so mamma cow does not need to say twice, "Help yourself!"

The baby calf is very glad to suck milk from its mother's breast until its teeth are full grown. Then it begins to eat hay, and grass and grain, and by and by it stops nursing entirely, to eat just what its mother eats.

As cows are very precious animals, they generally have but one calf at a time, although twin calves are sometimes seen. Most mares, or mamma horses, have only one baby colt at a time, because horses are very precious too, but cats often have four or five kittens at once, and dogs three or four puppies.

Because cats, and dogs, and pigs, have several babies to nurse at a time, God has given them several breasts, which fill with milk whenever the babies need it. In that way, all the babies can nurse at once, and have all the milk they want or need.

Baby cows and baby horses come into the world all covered with hair, and with wide open eyes; but puppies and kittens are not one bit pretty at first. Their eyes are tightly closed when born because they are not yet strong enough to bear the light. In about nine days they grow strong enough to open and then the puppies and kittens can see all right.

There are some children, who, not knowing what I have told you, actually try to open the eyes of poor little puppies or kittens! This is horribly cruel. It hurts the delicate little creatures so dreadfully, that they often become blind from it.

So, children, never, never handle little animal babies until you have learned all about them, for, without meaning to do so, you may do them more harm than you can imagine, and spoil all their happy lives.

QUESTIONS.—Is it always easy for fathers and mothers to explain all the things you want to know? What is the fairy-tale told to little children about Christmas, and what is the truth? What is "Nature's Secret," and with whom may you talk about it? When God made the first tree, plant, bit of grass, etc., what purpose was it to serve? Did God make all living things of two sexes, male and female, and why? Are there plant, animal, and human families? Do Father and Mother Flower always live in the same house? What do you see in the middle of every open flower? Tell the story of a flower family. Do all flowers and plants and trees grow from seeds? Where do fishes live, and is their blood colder or warmer than yours? What is fish-roe, and how does it turn into fishes? Tell the story of a bird family. Do all animals grow from seeds or eggs? Why should you be careful of little puppies and kittens?

CHAPTER XVI

How You Came Here

AFTER learning exactly how all the plant, fish, bird and animal babies come into the world, I suppose you wonder how you got here yourself. Since I promised to tell you all you care to know about yourself, I am going to tell you that too.

You know that you are very different from animals. They have bodies, and life, and instinct, but they have no mind or soul, such as you have. It is because you have a mind and a soul that you are said to be made after God's own image.

When you were little, you often asked where you came from, and as you could not understand then, what I am going to tell you now, you were probably told fairy-tales, or things which were only true in a way. Mamma may have told you that God sends all the little babies. That is perfectly true, for all life does come from God. You may also have seen pictures like this, where a lovely angel brings a laughing baby down from Heaven in its arms. But if you had really come to papa and mamma in this way, they could not love you quite as much as they do now, for the reason you are soon going to hear.

If your parents ever heard German fairy-tales, or if you had a

German nurse, you may have been told that a stork came flying in one day, carrying you in his bill, and that he laid you down beside mamma, and bit her leg, so that she had to stay in bed until quite well again. That too, is only a fairy-tale, like the story of Santa Claus. But it is great fun to believe it when you are too little to understand the truth.

You may also have been told that the doctor brought you, or that mamma found you in a cabbage, or something of the sort. There is a speck of truth about all these stories, as you will see when you know all.

You heard, did you not, how the male and female bird found each other and how they agreed to make a dear little home for themselves and for their family? Well, when a man is quite grown up, when he is strong and well, and feels that he can earn enough to make a home, he begins to think about marrying, too. As he has a soul, he wants to find a wife with a soul like his, a wife whom he can love and trust.

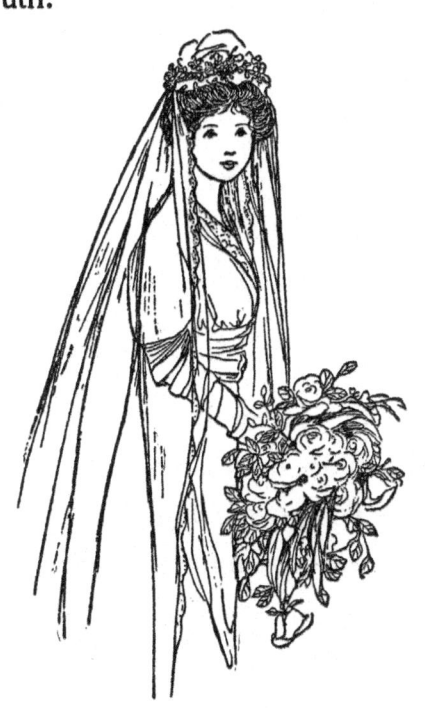

THE BRIDE

He looks around, and when he meets the right woman—the

woman who has a soul like his,—he asks her to be his wife, and come and make a home for him. Then they two are married, either by a priest or by a minister, if they are Christians or believe in any special religion, or before a magistrate, if they prefer.

In marrying, the man promises to love his wife, to work for her, to take care of her when she is sick and when she is well, and to be not only a good husband to her alone, but a good father to any children God may send into his home. You see, this is a very solemn promise. Because a good home is the loveliest thing in the world, every one feels interested in such a young couple, and all their friends wish them luck, health, and happiness, and bring them gifts.

How You Grew

You have all seen weddings, have you not? And you all know that when the wedding is over, it is right and proper for the young woman to leave her father and mother, and go away with the young man, so that they can begin a new life together, and make a new home. Never mind what kind of a home it is, whether it is in one small room only, or in the grandest palace you ever saw, if the man and woman really love each other, wherever they are together, they are at home, and they feel so strongly that they are one, that they often, in joking-earnest, talk of each other as their "better half."

At first, your family was a very small one, only papa and mamma. While father was away at work all day, mother was quite alone, and when she saw other homes where there were little children to keep the mothers company, she often wished she had some too.

Mamma knew that the souls of people (the masters of their little houses), are sent by God, to live in human bodies. Although she did not know what souls are made of—nobody does know that except God,—she knew that the little houses in which they live and grow are made of food and air.

Mamma knew that in her body, just as in the body of all female animals, there was a little room which God made as a home for tiny babies. In that room, mamma's little blood-boats made a tiny little egg, so small that it could not be seen except with a microscope. Just like the bird's egg, it grew and changed as soon as some of father's life fluid got into it.

But this tiny egg was hatched inside of mother's body, and when you first came out of it, you were so small, so very small, that no one could have seen you. Babies as small as that could not of course be handled at all, so God decided that they should stay right in the little room where they were hatched, until big enough to be trusted out in this world. Just so, baby birds are kept *in the nest* until it is safe for them to leave it.

You, therefore, stayed in mother's little room, week after week and month after month, for about three-quarters of a year. Mother knew you were there, for she could feel your little hand or foot tapping against the wall of the room as if to say, "how do you do" to her. Mother could not see you, and did not know what you looked like, but she could *feel* you were alive—just as you can feel your heart beat—and she knew that you were growing. As you were part of mother's body and alive, you needed both food and air. These were brought to you by mother's blood-boats.

Mother wanted her baby to be as well and strong as possible, so she was very careful to breathe nice pure air, and to eat nothing but good wholesome food. She also wanted you to grow as big as you could, so she did not wear any tight clothes at all, so as not to squeeze you up in that little room. Because she wanted you to be a jolly, happy baby, she thought only of nice, pleasant things, tried to be happy all the time, and sang and smiled while at work.

As long as you lived in the little room in mother's body, you were warm and snug and safe, and while mother watched carefully over you, father watched as carefully over her. Like the father bird I told you about, he got all she needed, kept her company whenever he could, cheered and encouraged her, and, knowing no feathers grow on human babies, earned money enough to get clothes, so that you would have all you needed when you came into this world, or were born, as it is called.

As you grew bigger and bigger, you needed more and more air and food, and mother's blood-boats were so busy feeding you, and helping you to grow big and strong, that they could not spare much food or air to keep mother herself well and strong. But mother loved you so dearly, that she wanted you to have the very best she could give you, and she did not care at all what happened to her, as long as she knew that you were all right.

How You Came into the World

Next time you take a bath, just look at the queer little hole in the middle of your belly or abdomen. While you lived in mother's little room, a pipe went right down into this little hole, and through this pipe the blood-boats sent by mamma's pumping dwarfs, carried food and air into your tiny body, to build it up bit by bit with the materials they brought.

All the good air mother breathed, helped to make your little house, and all the good food she ate was just so much building material for you. That is why children are so often told that they were found in cabbages, in carrots, or in potatoes. Really, you know, the cabbages, carrots, potatoes, etc., only served to make a part of the blood out of which your little body was made.

There are some things—as I told you before—which no one has ever been able to find out. One of these is just when and how your soul got into your body. No one—not even the wisest doctor who ever lived—knows anything about this. But we believe that the soul was sent by God to live and grow in the little house which mother was so busy making for you.

When you were big enough to make it safe for you to come out into the world, God opened the door of the little room where you had been so snug and safe. Then you first saw the light, and mamma, who had been far more patient even than the mother bird I have told you about, was very, very happy to see and hear you at last.

As long as you lived in mamma's body, she breathed for you, but when you came out of the little room, the air rushed into your lungs, which now began their life work, and after that, you could, if necessary, have lived without mamma.

Sometimes, when God opens the door of the little room, the pain is so great, that poor mammas die, and as it always makes mothers very ill, the doctor generally has to come and take care of them. It is also the doctor who ties up the pipe opening in a baby's abdomen, and that is why mamma and nurses so often tell children that the baby came when the doctor did, and children fancy that he brought it in his satchel!

The little room in mamma's body where you lived before you were born is made of soft skin, and is warm and moist just like the inside of your mouth. Put your finger in your mouth and just leave it there for awhile, closing your lips tightly over it. When you take it out again, you will find that it is much warmer and redder than the other fingers, and slightly wrinkled. Now, you know, *you* stayed in the little room—where it was so warm and so moist—for many, many months, so it is no wonder that when you came out first, you were very red and wrinkled.

Many people when they first see a new-born baby are terribly disappointed because it is red and wrinkled, but now you know just why it is so. In a few days the wrinkles go away, baby is no longer as red as a little lobster, and then you can see how pretty it really is.

Little babies are so delicate, that mammas and nurses have to take the very best care of them. No cold air must strike them at first, no bright light shine in their weak eyes, no loud noises startle them, and no rough touch hurt them. But, as mother is often too ill to look after the baby at first, she often has some one else to help her; still, as soon as she gets well enough, she generally takes care of her dear baby her own self.

WHY YOU SHOULD LOVE YOUR MOTHER

As little babies,—like all birds and other animals,—need plenty of food to grow, and as they cannot as yet eat the same kind of food we do, God sends milk into mother's breasts to feed them. But if mother is not very strong, she sometimes finds that she has not milk enough to satisfy her baby, and then she gives it a bottle.

Because mothers give a part of their own life to their children, because they have to watch over them so long before they come, and because they often suffer such pain when they are born, mothers love them much more than if they came straight down from Heaven in an angel's arms.

You know how it is yourself, you always like even a doll or a toy better when it is all your own, than when you buy it in a store or if it is given to you. So mamma loves her baby much better than any other because it is her very own.

Good mothers feel that God is very kind when He lets them have a baby of their very own, and sends down a little soul to dwell in its tiny body. They know that the time will come when the body will die, but they feel that the soul will never die, and they want to make it beautiful and strong so they can tell God that they carefully trained the soul He trusted to their keeping.

It is because mother has done so much for you—so much more than you can ever understand, until you are a father or mother yourself,—that you ought always to love her, to obey her, and to be as good to her as you can. No boy or girl can ever be too good to his or her mother, nor too ready to help or to serve her. When she grows old and you grow up, you must always remember that it is your turn now to take care of her, and thus repay her a little, for all she has done for you.

Whenever we see a boy or girl loving and obedient, trying to help his or her mother and to please her, we know that she is a proud and happy mother, and we feel sure that her child will turn into a good man or woman.

When we see a boy rude to his mother, or disobedient, we think: "Either you have no idea of what your mother suffered for you, and of all she did for you, or you are a little brute!"

When a girl lets her mother do all the work, and thinks of nothing but her own comfort or pleasure, we think: "If you

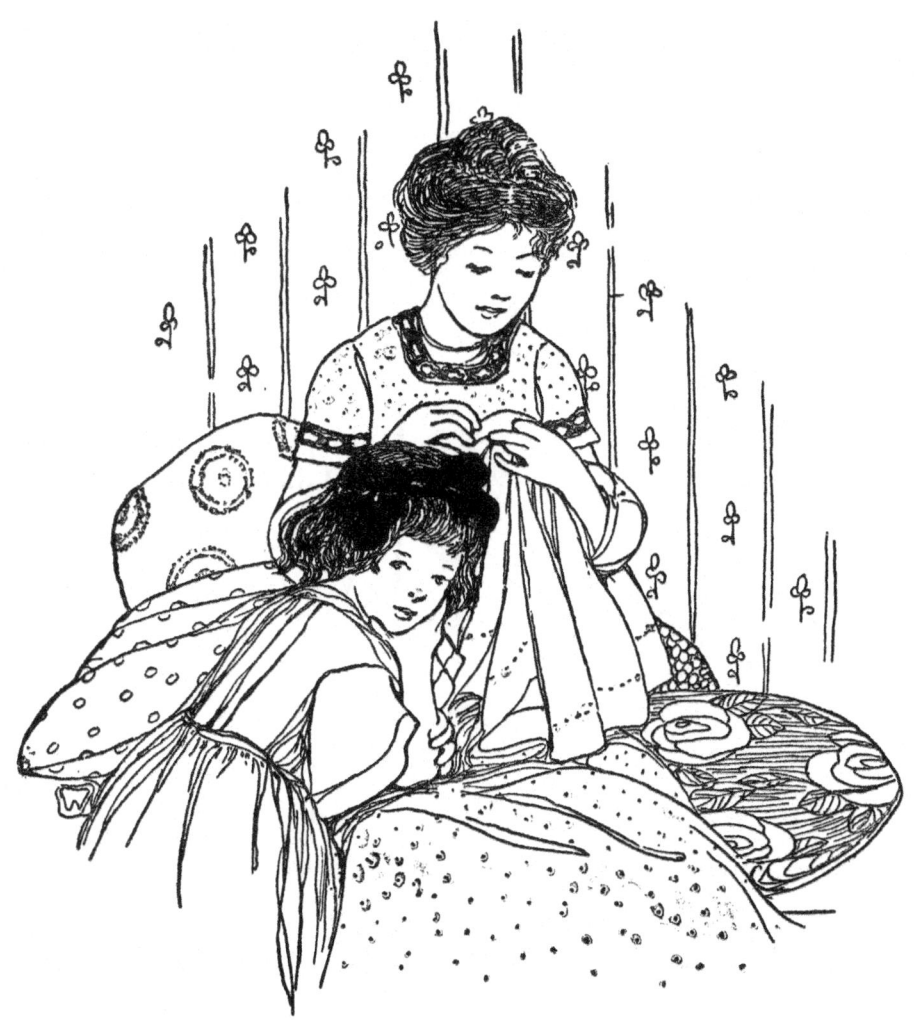

TRY TO PLEASE MOTHER ALWAYS

know how your mother cared for you, before you came into the world, and while you were a wee baby, you are an ungrateful little wretch if you do not help her now, for you should be only too glad to be able to do something for her in your turn."

Why You Should Love Your Father

We have talked a great deal about your mother until now, but remember that your father has a share in you too. Because he gave you life, because he took care of you and of mother all the time you were growing, because he gave you the clothes you wear, and the food you eat, because he helped take care of you while you were helpless, and gives you a home, you ought to love him very dearly and obey him just as well as mother.

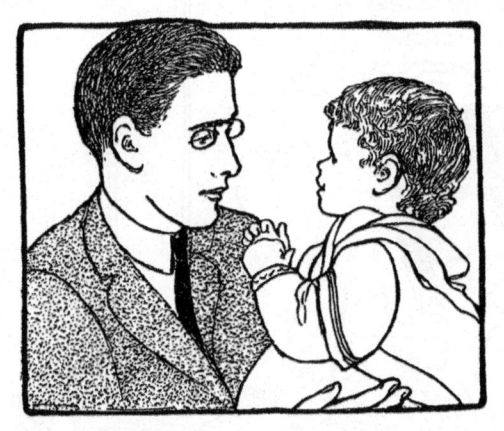

FATHER WANTS TO FEEL PROUD OF YOU

Remember that good fathers and mothers are watching their children all the time. If you grow up to be the kind of man or woman of whom they can be proud, they will be so happy! But if you bring shame upon them, if you are idle or disobedient, you will make them very, very unhappy. Just think how glad you will feel if they can say every year: "I am so glad you were born, you have always been such a blessing to your father and mother!" But just imagine too how badly you would feel, if you knew that they wished you had never been born! Good husbands and fathers, and all real gentlemen are always very kind to their wives and children, for they know how easily they can be hurt for life, and no man or boy who knows how tender a woman's body is, or what harm a blow can do her, ever dreams of laying a rough hand upon her. Indeed any one who will strike a woman is rightly considered a great brute.

When older people see a woman walking heavily or looking rather large, they think: "This may be a woman whom God is honoring. Perhaps He is entrusting to her the care of an immortal soul." Then they feel they cannot do too much for her; so, wherever she goes, she is sure to find good men and women ready to help her, and to give her a seat in a car or on a boat. They show her all respect for the sake of their own dear mothers, who, while they were coming into the world, needed all the care and tenderness that could be shown to them.

Never be rude therefore, children, or make unkind remarks. What you call a "fat woman," *may* be a woman who gave up all her good looks and health for her children's sake, or perhaps she may be a woman "with child," as the Bible says, in speaking of women whose little babies have not yet been born.

About Sex

I have explained to you already that as I am telling you all about your own body I often have to speak of private things,

things which are not mentioned as a rule. But I expect you to show your sense by acting like little men or women, and not like silly imps. *Nice* children will read all I have to tell them in this book without giggling, or nudging each other, and they certainly will not speak about the sacred parts of this book to any one save their mother.

You *may* think now that you can speak to any one about it, but if you do, you will be very sorry when you grow old enough to understand that there are some matters too intimate and too sacred to be talked about lightly.

If you do not want to be very, very sorry, and feel the blush of shame rise to your cheek every time you think of what you have done, you will keep your mouth very tightly shut now, and you will stop your ears, and run away, if any one but mother, father or teacher tries to talk about these matters to you. Those who do so, are either so ignorant that they do not even know that these are strictly private matters, or they are so evil-minded that you must have nothing to do with them. Now that I have warned you again, I think it is safe to go on teaching you what it is right that you should know.

The very first question every one asks when they hear that a new baby has come, is: "Is it a boy or a girl?" You see, it is God only who decides who may have babies, and of what sex or kind they shall be. There are many, many fathers and mothers who would like to have babies, but God does not let them. Why that is so, nobody knows, but those who trust and love God, believe that He has some very good reason, although they do not know it.

There is another thing which none of us can understand very well, that is why God sometimes sends such precious things as little babies to bad or careless people. Perhaps it is because He thinks that is the only way in which to make them good once more.

Even your papa and mamma—who knew so long beforehand that a baby was coming to their house—had no idea just when you would appear, and whether you would be a boy or a girl. Baby boys and baby girls are just alike in everything, except their private parts, and it was only when you came into this world naked, that the very first glance showed them to what sex you belonged. God makes babies different, because they are to grow up differently into men or into women.

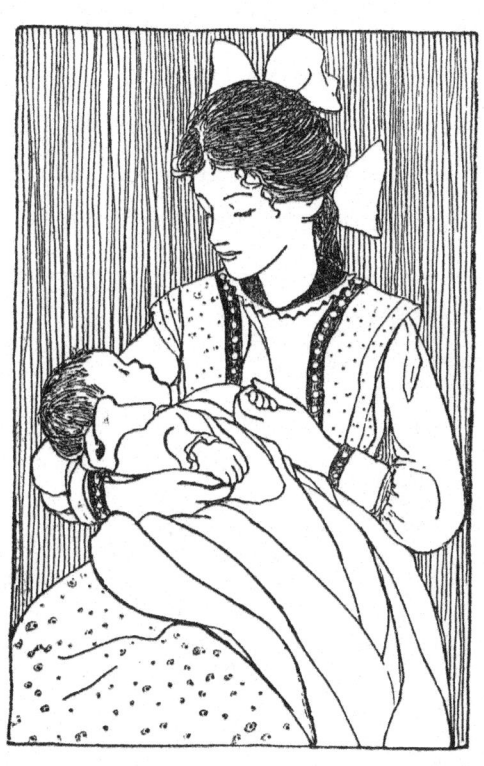

THE BABY SISTER

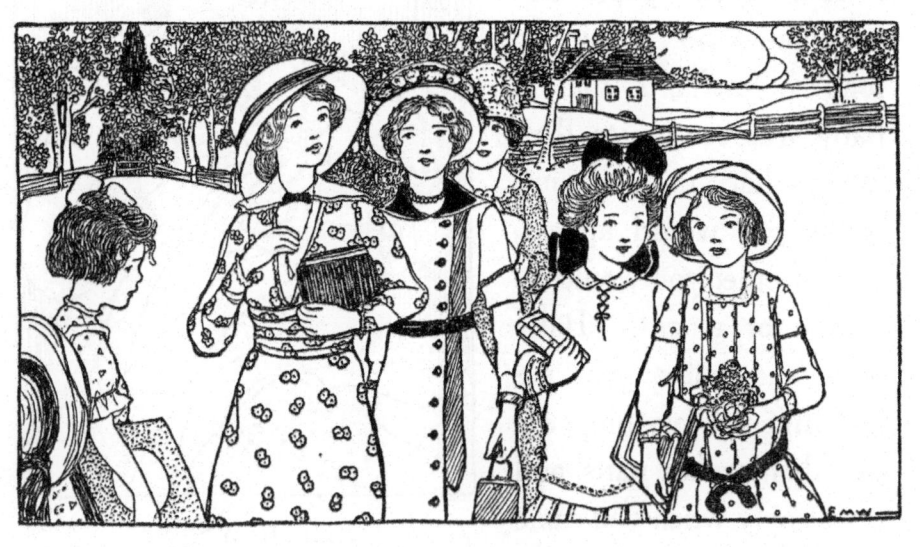

The Seven Year Periods

During the first seven years—the years of babyhood as they are often called,—boys and girls cut all their first set of teeth, grow from soft little babies into sturdy youngsters, and learn ever so many things. Doctors often tell us that it takes just about seven years for the blood-boats to renew every part of our body according to the pattern God gave them. This is why we often divide life up into seven year periods.

During the next seven years—the time of girlhood and of boyhood—children grow almost as fast as before, learn a great

The Seven Year Periods

deal more, and cut their second teeth. All their body is new again, but still they are exactly the same, scars and all, and so is the Master of their little house.

The next seven years are called the "teens" or youth. During that time boys and girls grow into men and women, and generally they finish their school life.

During their "teens" we see them grow taller and broader, more wise and more thoughtful, the boys' voices change, and the girls' forms grow rounder, and by these signs all grown people know that nature is finishing her work, and little by little turning these children into men and women.

Fathers and mothers always feel a little sorry to see them grow so fast, because they know that as children grow older the duties of life will rest more and more heavily upon their young shoulders.

During the fourth period of seven years, men and women are full grown, and ready to begin to make homes of their own if they choose to do so. If they have been wise, and have treated their bodies in the right way, they are as straight and strong and healthy as they can be. If they have treated their minds in the right way too, their brain storehouse is packed with good and useful things, and their muscles and nerves are trained to work as quickly and neatly as a first-class machine. Such men and women can make good homes, and bring up wisely the children God gives them.

By the time fathers and mothers reach the fifth, sixth, and seventh period of seven years and begin to feel a little tired, their children are generally old enough to wait on them a little, to run errands for them, and to save them in many ways. We are told that men or women are old only when they have reached seventy years of age, but many people live to be ninety and even one hundred years old if they do not abuse their bodies.

QUESTIONS.—In what are you different from animals? What are the fairy-tales told about babies? What does a man promise when he marries? What makes a real home? Were you too small to be born at first, and where did mamma keep your little body? Where did your soul come from? Did mother know you would come out of the little room some day, and how did she prepare to welcome you? How did mother feed you in the little room? About how long did you stay in mother's little room? Why are new born babies red, wrinkled and very tender? When did you begin breathing for yourself? How were you fed after you were born? Has mother been very good to you? How should you repay your mother for all she has done for you? What does a father do for his children? Ought you to love and obey him just as well as you love and obey your mother? What kind of a boy or girl is a blessing to his or her parents? How do all rightly-minded people consider any man or any boy who strikes a woman or a girl? Who decides into what families babies shall go, and whether they shall be boys or girls? How often do the blood-boats renew your whole body, what is the first period called, and why? What is the second period called, and what teeth do you cut? What are the teens, and what change takes place in your house while they last? What can you tell about the other seven-year periods, and the length of human lives?

CHAPTER XVII

How to Grow Rightly

JUST look at the picture opposite page 300. Do you see this dear little girl thinking only of her flowers, and picking more to add to the bunch she holds? Do you see this little boy trying to catch a butterfly even on the edge of a deep precipice?

These children know so little about danger, that they have wandered to the very edge of this abyss. One step further, and they would surely fall over, and be dashed to pieces. But they are such very little children, so young and so ignorant, that God has sent an angel to watch over them. The angel has his hands stretched over them, ready to catch them and hold them back from harm.

It is nice, is it not, to see that angel so near those happy children and to know that no harm can happen to the dear little things, although they are in such a dangerous place!

As long as you were very little, mother was always there to save you from harm, to hold her hand between you and any sharp corner of the furniture so that you should not get a bad bump or cut, and to guard you night and day.

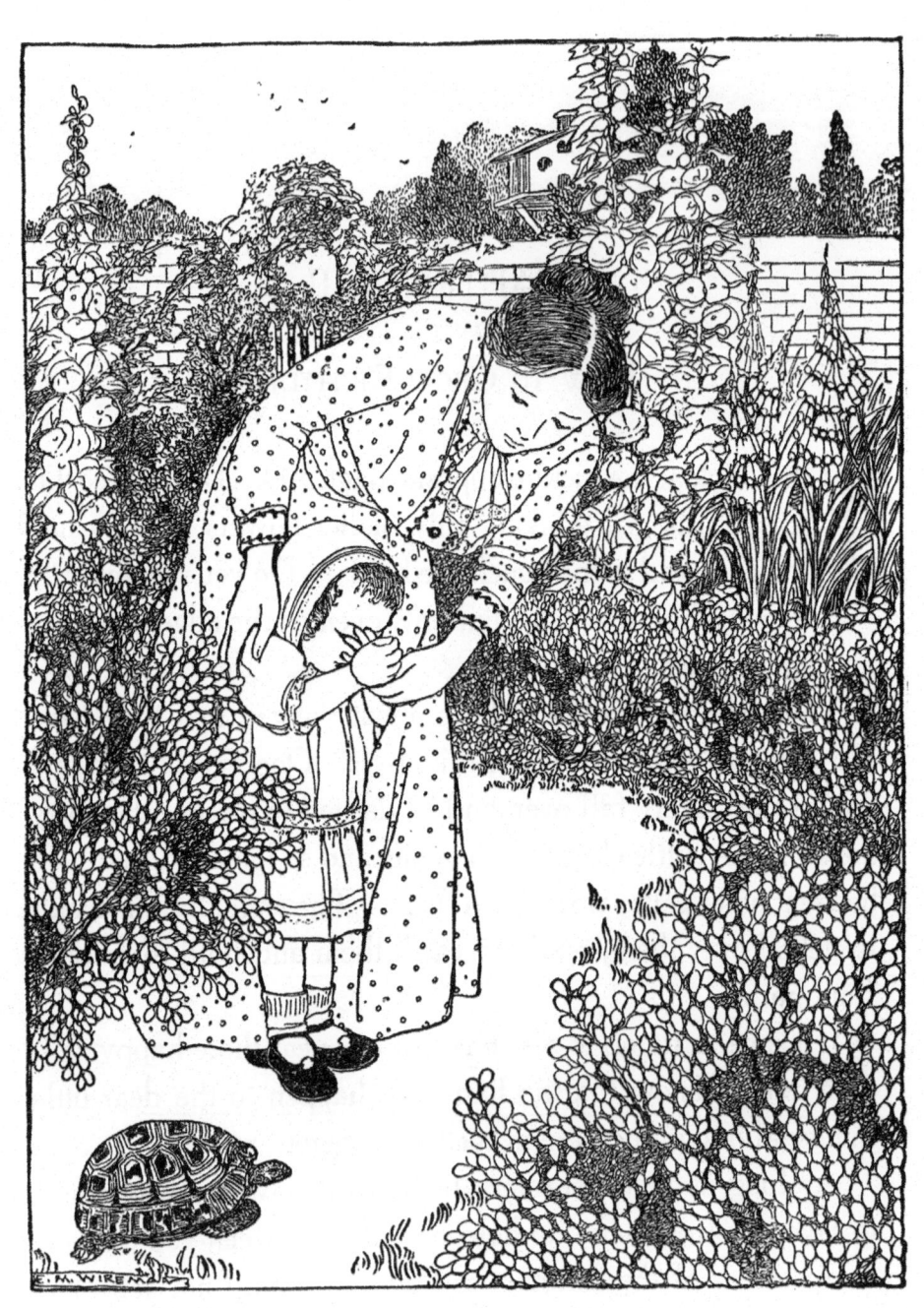

MOTHER GUARDS YOU FROM HARM

How to Grow Rightly

Now that you are older, mother cannot go with you everywhere. She cannot warn you every time you come to dangerous places, and cannot snatch you away from harm. But if you live in the country, she tells you, for instance, not to go too near the pond, where the water is deep, and if you live in the city, never to cross the street when a trolley car is coming. Still, she knows that the master in your house must look out for you now, and be your guardian angel.

Your teachers also warn you of all kinds of dangers. They warn you, for instance, of the danger of telling lies, of being dishonest, of growing lazy or selfish, and of many others. Now there is another danger which you must all be warned against,—that of losing your purity, both of body and mind.

You know the difference, do you not, between a glass of pure water and a glass of dirty water? Which would you rather have to drink? There is the same difference—only it is much greater,—between pure and impure minds and pure and impure bodies. All well-meaning people, long to have and to keep their bodies and minds as pure as they can; but, to have them pure and keep them pure, they must know just what that means.

You remember how you learned, in the middle of this book, that every thought we think, every word we hear, everything we see and learn is stored away in our brain—whether we know it or not,—and that it can never be changed or rubbed out?

If you think only nice, pure, noble thoughts, those only will be stored away in your brain; but if you think horrid, impure, mean thoughts, it will be those which will soon fill up your brain storehouse. You must, therefore, be very careful what company you keep, what books you read, what you say and what you do, for all that makes up what you are.

Girls and boys who read only about pirates, fights, murders, thefts, and adventures of an exciting kind, store away in their brain all the mean, ugly and horrible things they read. Now, you surely don't want to grow up to be thieves, murderers, or other vile wretches, do you? Then why are you storing away in your brain all the sayings and doings of such folks?

If you want to grow up to be a hero or heroine, read about all the fine, strong, noble things you can. By and by, when the time comes, you will know what the grand people of the world did, and little by little, you will build up a character like theirs, and perhaps thus learn to do things even greater than any they ever did.

How to Keep Pure

To keep our souls and minds pure and noble in this way is the very best thing we can do, but to do that we must also keep our bodies clean and pure. I have explained how to keep your *skin* clean, but it is something more than that which I mean by bodily purity.

I am going to try to explain it to you, however hard it may

How to Keep Pure

be, so that you can understand it clearly. When bodies are beautiful, and strong and healthy, and all that they should be, we agreed that instead of merely being called houses, they really deserved the grander name of temple.

When you come to study history, you will hear of the grandest temple the world has ever seen, which once stood in Jerusalem. This temple was a huge building, decorated with marble, and gold, and precious stones. It was built by God's order, and that temple was called His house.

People who wanted to worship God went into this temple, where there were many courts and many rooms. In some of these rooms strangers were allowed to enter, in others the worshippers, in others the priests and no one else. In the most secret and safest part of the temple there was a little place, which was called the Holy of Holies, which no one was allowed to enter.

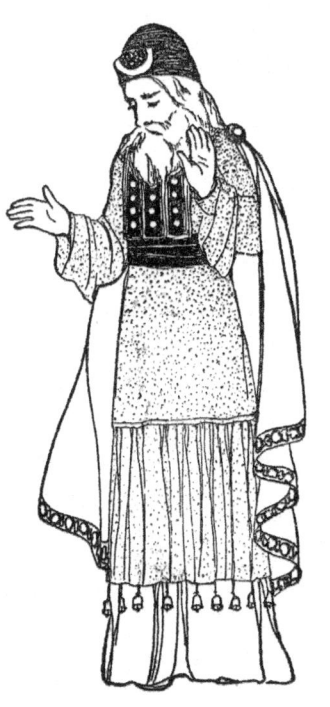

THE HIGH PRIEST

This was such a sacred place, that no one could come near it, nor was any one allowed to lay as much as a finger on the big curtain which cut it off from the rest of the temple. Once a year, after he had said many prayers and done many other things, the High Priest went into this place by God's order. He could enter only then, and only if he had done just as God wished.

As long as this place was kept sacred in this way, the temple stood and was fine and beautiful. But there was a war. Some soldiers came into the temple. They were wicked men who respected nothing. They raised the curtain, and went into the Holy of Holies, and—to show how little they cared for the people who built it, or for God,—they drove pigs right into this sacred place!

The Holy of Holies, which had been kept so pure and clean until then, was no longer pure and clean, and because God wanted this to be forever after a lesson to all the world, He allowed that beautiful temple to be destroyed. All the worth and the beauty of it was gone, because it was no longer pure and sacred.

Now, as I told you, it rests with us to make temples of our bodies if we choose. God has put into each human body a sacred little place which is the body Holy of Holies. He wishes us to keep it pure, to keep it well hidden (our clothes are the curtain), and to guard it against any impure thought or touch.

In a man's body, this Holy of Holies is the place where the life fluid or seed is made; and in the woman's body, it is the little room which God made as a nest for babies. The place where the seed is made is in man's private parts, and the door of every woman's little room opens in the same passage as the one which empties the waste water.

As long as we remember that these parts of our body are holy, and keep them pure, all is well; but, if we are careless, if we forget, or if we are wicked, we lose our bodily purity, or our bodily honor, and our body is no longer a temple.

How Boys and Girls Become Men and Women

You know that a boy's voice does not change in a day from childish treble to a deep bass, and that a little girl takes some time to turn into a young woman. During that time the blood-boats are very busy. You see, they have to supply food and air enough to all your muscles to keep them going, and they have to make your house much bigger and broader in every way.

They work as hard as they can, but there is so much to do that sometimes they cannot supply food, air and materials enough. Then boys and girls are apt to feel cross, tired, lazy, and languid; they often feel like crying when there is nothing really to cry about, and they are generally uncomfortable and unhappy.

If you feel that way while in your "teens," just be patient with yourself. Remember that before long your blood-boats will manage to do all the work your body needs. Then you will grow cheerful and strong again and all will we well. But, if you fret, if you pity yourself, if you don't try to control those feelings as much as you can, you will meantime be storing away ever so many fretful, complaining, weak-minded cells in your brain storehouse, and then you cannot grow into a hero or heroine, unless you learn to conquer those bad habits.

Every boy and girl during his or her teens—when he or she is laying the foundations for a strong man or woman—or for a weakling—ought to be particularly careful to consult often the three greatest doctors the world has ever seen, that is to say Dr. Water, Dr. Diet and Dr. Exercise. If *their* orders are closely followed, the result will be good, if not,—well—no one will regret it more than you.

All during their teens, girls should be particularly careful to live wisely and not to wear tight clothes. You already know what mischief tight clothes do to many parts of the body at all times, but while you are changing into a woman, they can cramp that little room, and by hurting it, make all the little nerves which connect it with the rest of the body very, very sore and sick.

How to Care for Certain Parts of the Body

You remember, do you not, how I told you there were many nerves in the body? Well, the most delicate ones run from your private parts up to your brain, spine, and all the other parts of your body.

If the private parts are always kept very clean, by frequent

How to Care for Certain Parts of the Body 285

and careful washings, and always handled gently while doing so, no harm will be done to these delicate nerves. But if the private parts are not kept clean, if they are roughly handled, or if the clothes press too tightly upon them, those nerves will get very weak and will make the whole body unhappy. Now you understand, do you not, why you must be so careful even of a baby, and why you should always prevent your little brothers or sisters from touching their private parts.

It is not all to be careful with very little children. Every human being has to be careful about this as long as life lasts. The older you grow, the more careful you *must* be, for if these parts are roughly treated, or handled at all when not needful, you can lose your health and strength and even your mind.

That is why your mammas try to train you from the very first never to touch this part of your person except when you must, to keep it clean, and to be modest at all times, and keep it always covered. Any boy or girl who is not careful about this, at all times, is *not* a nice child, and you must avoid all such just as if they had the smallpox.

You have probably heard, time and again in your lives, that boys are made of "hobs and nails and puppy dog tails," while girls are made of "sugar and spice and all things nice." Of course, that is only a nonsense rhyme, for boys and girls are really made of exactly the same things.

But, you are told this, because fathers and mothers want you boys to learn as soon as possible to handle girls very gently; and as you could not understand the truth when little, you were told in a nonsense way. Until ten, a girl often minds hard knocks just as little as a boy, but after that, while a boy's body daily grows harder, hers grows softer. A touch which he would not feel, actually hurts her.

Besides, there is one part of every woman's body which is very sensitive, and where the least little blow often causes great pain. This is in the breast. Many women feel shy about saying anything about it, because as they know what God made the breasts for, they feel they are too sacred to mention.

Until God sends milk into the breasts to feed newborn babies, they are very delicate, and I believe that many women wear corsets mainly because they serve to protect this tender place in their bodies.

BOYS SHOULD BE GENTLE WITH GIRLS

Many growing boys have no idea how strong they are getting, how long their arms are, and how tough their fingers. They grab at their sisters, just as they used to do when they were little girls. The sisters—who are often hurt so badly that they have to go away and cry—then scream, and the boys say scornfully, "Oh! girls are always squealing!" but the fact is that if any one hurt those very boys half as badly, they would surely thrash that person!

The bigger and stronger you get, boys, the gentler you have to learn to be to all the women and children, not only in your own family, but everywhere else. God gave you all that size and strength so that you could protect women and children, but remember you must always protect them *first* against any roughness or unkindness from yourselves.

ABOUT KISSING

At school, at church, and in many of the good books you will read, you will hear and see over and over that it is the duty of every man and woman, and of every boy and girl, not only to be as healthy as possible, but to keep their minds and bodies pure. You now know exactly what that means, and I trust you all mean to take it to heart.

Of course, you have already found out that *all* books are not good, and that there are some very bad people in this world. You know, for instance, that some swear, some lie, some steal, some murder, and it is true also, that some do not care at all about keeping either their minds or their bodies pure.

As I told you before, all pure-minded people—who look upon their bodies as a temple which must be kept holy—feel that love, and marriage, and babies, are just as sacred in their way as their religion.

Little children, who do not know any better, often play church, pretend to say prayers, and talk about God as if He were just like themselves. But older children, who have learned that church, prayers and God are sacred subjects, never dream of playing at anything of the sort.

In the same way, little children, and people who have no real respect for themselves or for others, can play at love and marriage. In little children this is not wrong—for they do not know any better and their play means nothing,—but in older people, who ought to feel that there is something too sacred about it for play, it is often very, very wrong.

Boys and girls who are in a great hurry to grow up, often think they will appear older if they ape the manners of their elders. So, the boys put on lover-like airs, and the girls turn sentimental and try to flirt. If all this were not so very foolish and silly, that all parents know that the really sensible boys and girls will soon see it and stop it themselves, they would check it right away.

Many parents do warn their daughters that there is nothing they will feel more sorry for when they grow up, than if they have allowed a lot of boys to treat them in a lover-like way. How would you like to be called by them a "pawed over girl" for instance? And people will call you that very thing, if you allow men and boys to flirt with you, and hug and kiss you.

After a little girl gets to be ten, and grows into girlhood, she ought to feel that she is too old to be treated like a baby. Nice girls of that age cannot bear to be kissed or hugged by any one except the men and boys in their own family.

Perhaps, when they were babies, all their father's friends got into the habit of kissing and hugging them. Such men often do not realize that little girls grow big, although they may remark how tall they are getting. When they offer to kiss you, it is perfectly right and proper for you to say: "Please excuse me. I am no longer a baby now, and I would much rather shake hands with you, if you don't mind."

Any gentleman, who is not a dreadful tease, will respect even a little girl's wishes in such matters, and even the worst tease that ever lived, will stop if you show him plainly that you are really in earnest. Any man or boy who tries to kiss you, in spite of your telling him you do not wish it, is *ungentlemanly,* and if he kisses you by force, after you have warned him not to do so, he deserves to be punished. I would therefore advise every girl in the United States, if she cannot run away, to slap such a man right in the face, and to slap him hard!

Tattle-tales are, as we know, very silly people, but if any one bothers you about this, it is right and proper for you to make a fuss, and to complain to your father, to your mother, or to your brothers. But if, in a game, with many people all around you, some one should happen to kiss you, just take it as a matter of course, and if you dislike it, all you need do is not to take part in such games hereafter.

Never allow any one outside of your own family to kiss you on the mouth. If you do, you are likely to catch any cold or disease that person may have, for people are often sick before they know it themselves. For that reason, no one should ever

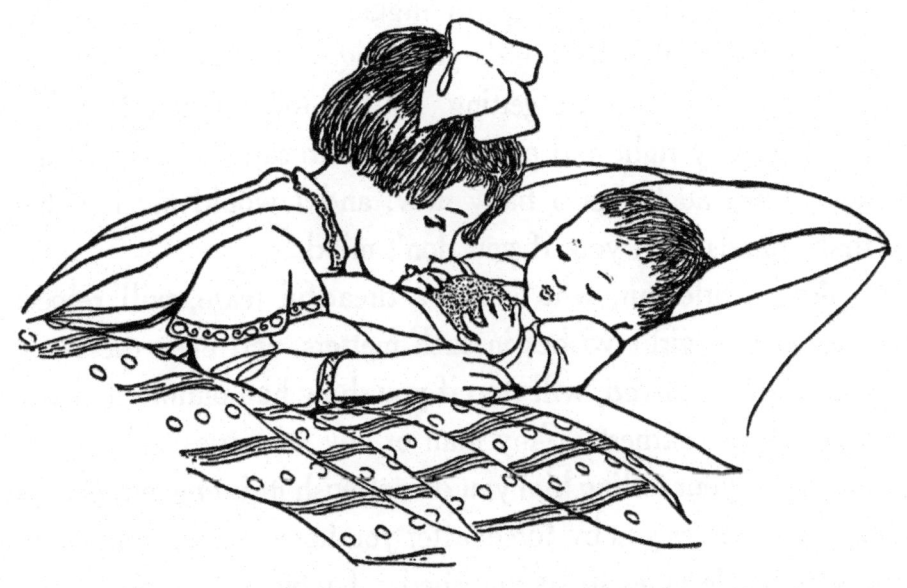

DON'T KISS BABY ON THE LIPS

kiss a baby on the lips. Babies do not like it and the people who kiss them so, torment them, and are selfish.

Any girl who shows by all her actions that she always respects herself, is sure sooner or later to win everybody's respect. Of course, you may be called prim, and stiff, and a prude, at

About Kissing 291

first, but such names never do a girl any harm at all, while to be called a flirt, a coquette, or worse still, *fast,* is very bad indeed. Many good people think that such a girl is either very vulgar and badly brought up, or that she has neither a pure soul nor a pure body.

QUESTIONS.—Who must watch over you all your life to see you form good habits? Is it right to be truthful, read good books, think nice thoughts, do kind deeds? What was the Holy of Holies in the Temple of Jerusalem, and how was it made impure? As each human body is a Temple for the spirit God sent to live there, should its Holy of Holies be kept pure and clean? Should you be particularly careful during your teens of your health and of the cleanliness of certain parts of your body? Are all people good, and do all consider their bodies holy and keep them as healthy and pure as they can? Are love, marriage, and babies sacred to all good people? Is it right for girls and boys to play at love? Is it right for girls to allow men and boys outside of the family to hug and kiss them? Is it right to kiss babies on the lips?

CHAPTER XVIII

Your Companions

MANY of you children have to leave home and school very early, and go into stores and shops, where some of you will meet rough and bad men and women. You will then hear bad language of all kinds, for all the wicked people talk very freely. They will, perhaps, even try to talk to you about sacred things in a nasty way, and will make fun of you for being good.

Mind all this as little as you can. All boys and girls with strong characters, come out of these trials all the better and stronger. They are "gold tried in the fire," and if they come out pure, it proves that they are really good metal.

If you are firm and true, if you stick to what you know or feel to be right, if you shut your ears and your mind, as much as you can, to all the wrong around you, the good people—and there are some good ones everywhere—will stand by you and help you.

The only trouble with good people is that many of them are often too timid, too afraid of hurting other people's feelings. There are, for instance, any number of men, who know that men and women should be equally careful of their purity, but who are quite satisfied to keep good themselves, and to avoid all those who do not think as they do.

In one way they are right, we should never keep bad company; but really brave men never allow any base or low talk or doings to go on in their presence. They are always ready to stand up for the right, and to use all their strength and influence to protect other men, women, and children from harm.

Always believe what such good men tell you, and do not listen to any man or boy who says that it makes no difference if a young man does "sow wild oats"—or do things which his conscience tells him are wrong. Men who talk like that, have either never given any serious thought to this matter, or they are bad, in spots at least, themselves.

Girls in their teens cannot be too careful what company they frequent, nor can they keep too close to mother. Some foolish girls think that if a young man or boy is clean, nicely dressed, and well mannered, he must be a gentleman. But it is not always so. There are, for instance, many idlers who lounge about our streets. They may *look* like gentlemen, but it is often the case that all the dirty looking workmen who pass them are much more gentlemanly than they.

Such idlers often linger around, on purpose to talk to young and innocent girls. They flatter them, tease them, get them excited, and then go off to repeat what these thoughtless girls have said to their evil-minded friends, who twist the most innocent remarks around into meaning something very different, and far worse than you or I can imagine.

If you think such things cannot be true, just read this verse, and see how different the meaning of exactly the same words can be, if you change *only* the punctuation.

>There is a lady in our land
>Who has ten nails on every hand,
>Five and twenty on hands and feet,
>All this is true and no deceit.

This, as you see, is a very queer and wrong statement. But, rightly punctuated, it reads:

>There is a lady in our land
>Who has ten nails, on every hand
>Five, and twenty on hands and feet,
>All this is true and no deceit.

This is perfectly true and still not a word has been changed.

Do you see now why girls should be careful? Do you understand why it is wiser you should stay at home? Do you see why we tell you it is unsafe for you to go out at night, unless you *must?* Now, do you realize how right it is if your parents are careful of you, and how ready you should be to help and not to hinder them?

About Books

If you wish to be a noble woman, don't read many love stories. Most of them are as bad for your mind as much candy is for your stomach. They may be very sweet and pure, but you know, even too much of the purest kind of sugar is bad for your liver, and too many of the sweetest books are bad for your mind.

Girls who read too many love stories in their teens, often get dreamy and sentimental. They *think* about things instead of *doing* things, and they *wish* for what they have not, instead of *making the best* of what they have. Besides, novels deal mostly with love and marriage, and you ought to think as little as possible about those subjects, until you are much older. Of course, there have been girls who were married very, very young, but that is not only foolish, but really very wrong.

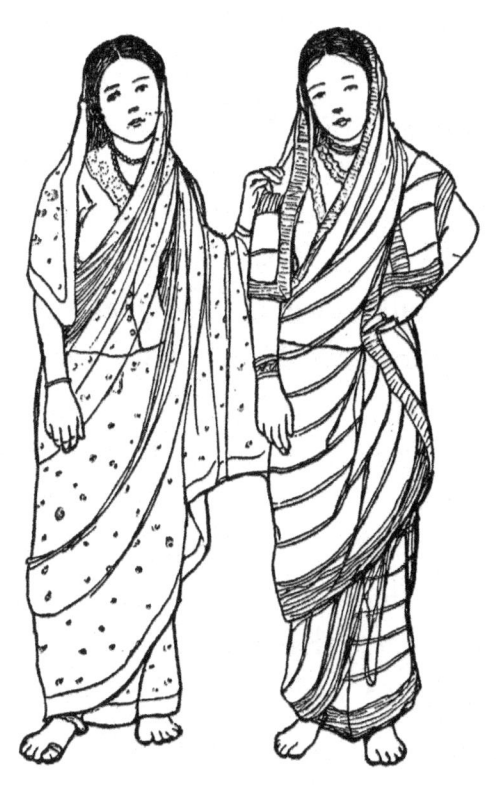

GIRLS OF INDIA

Girls in India, even now, often marry at twelve or thirteen, but what is the result? Travelers tell us that they have seen old, old women, bent and gray, and that when they inquired how old these women were, they found out that they were only thirty! Why, most women here are still very young at that age, and ever so many consider that it is hardly right to marry earlier, because they don't feel wise enough yet to bring up children.

The law, which allows people to marry just as soon as it is safe for them to do so, says that boys under twenty-one, and girls under eighteen, have not the right to marry without the consent of their parents. But all sensible young people realize, without any law, that they have no right to marry until they are full grown, and as a man's bones are never full size until he is about twenty-five, most men know it is not wise to marry sooner.

Besides, by that time, young men have generally learned what work they can do, how much they can earn, and if they are thrifty, they have also set aside part of their earnings, so that they can provide good homes for the wives who will be willing to share them.

Every boy or girl who hopes some day to be a good man or woman, will be good friends with the other girls and boys he or she meets, but will *not* do any courting or flirting. You can really have just as good, or even a better time, without doing so, and then you are sure not to have anything to regret.

About Pictures

Do you remember what I told you about your eyes, about the photographs they take, and about the picture gallery in your brain? On all sides you will see many beautiful pictures, in your school-books, in your homes, in the shop-windows, and in many of the magazines. All the nice and pretty pictures, and all the good ones, are fine to store away in your picture gallery.

But, just as there are good and bad books, there are also good and bad pictures. Now, many good people who know that purity is the finest thing in the world, think that all pictures and statues, showing people without clothes on, must be very wrong.

That is not so. Some are wrong and some are not. Long, long ago, people were just as good as they are now, and yet they did not wear any clothes at all. In fact, they did not need any, either to help them keep their bodies pure or to keep them warm. In hot countries, even now, few clothes are worn by the very young people, and many children never wear any at all, yet no one thinks any more of it than we do of seeing our baby naked.

There are also countries where women always keep their faces covered, yet do not care one bit if the rest of their body is seen. Clothes, you see, are mostly a matter of habit and custom. It is the custom here to wear a certain kind of garments, so, of course, people follow that custom.

An artist—who studies a long, long time before he becomes really skilled,—soon finds out that there is nothing more difficult to paint, to draw, to model, or to carve, than the human figure. He finds that it takes more knowledge of art and of science to paint the leg and foot of the little angel on the opposite page,—for instance—than to paint all the big angel's dress, the clouds and the city beneath them.

Artists study so long, that they little by little find out all the beauty of the human body. Every curve, every dimple, every shadow means something to them.

Artists like to paint the human form, not only because they see all its beauty, and because they can best show their skill in doing so, but also because people's clothes change so much that pictures soon look old-fashioned and ridiculous.

So that a picture should be really beautiful it must be like our idea of what it is meant to represent. If the angel, opposite page 299, wore a tailor-made gown and had gloves on, the picture would lose nearly all its beauty. The artist might know how to paint gowns and gloves so well that they looked real, but yet, as they would be out of place there, they would *spoil* the picture.

If an artist is painting a portrait of a real person, he of course, represents that person with the clothes he or she used to wear. But, if he paints fancy pictures, he likes to choose subjects where he can show his skill, subjects which pleased people hundreds of years ago, which please them now, and which will please their descendants hundreds of years from now.

If you look at a beautiful statue or a painting, thinking of the body as a temple, and of the skill of the artist, you won't do as some silly, ignorant people do, giggle and snicker, or blush and

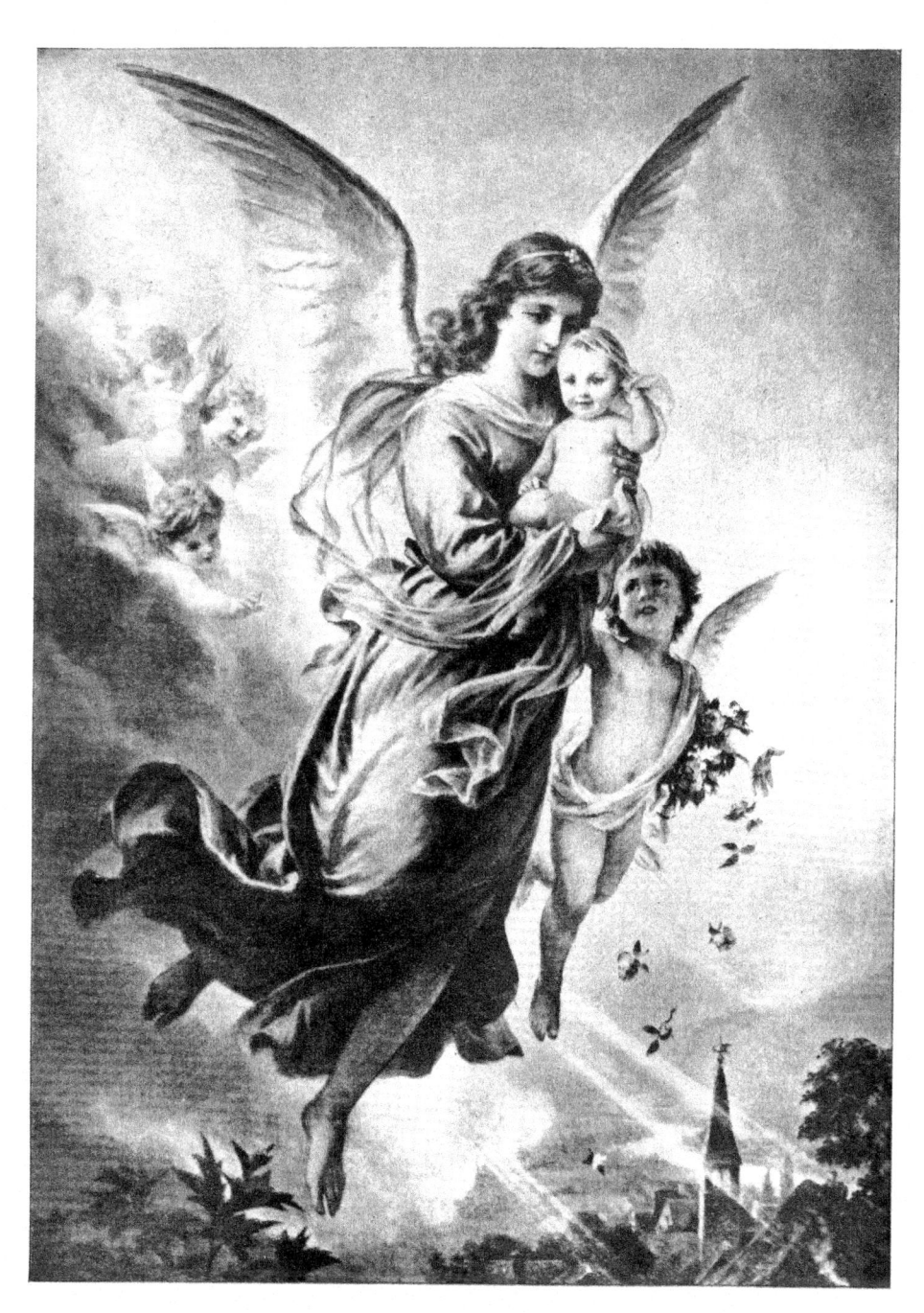

A Gift from Heaven

turn away your head simply because the human form is shown as God made it.

If you see a picture of a nude figure (one without clothes), look at it only to see the beauty of it. If the picture is a pure picture, and if *you* are pure yourself, you will like it more, the more you look at it, and you will have none but nice, pure thoughts about it.

If you are pure and the picture is not, the very first glance will be enough to make you feel a little uncomfortable, and you won't want to look at it again. Such pictures are never seen in really good books or magazines, or in nice picture stores. They are generally shown in places where pure-minded people never go, except by mistake, and then they get out again, as soon as possible, and never go back.

How to Get More Information

As you grow older, if you wish to know more about yourself than I could make you understand here,—although I have really told you all there is to tell,—get the books and magazines published by the Purity Society, or by any of your church societies. They will tell you nothing but what is right for you to know.

There are many other books on these subjects, but most of them are written by men who do not know what they are talking about, and who are trying only to make an easy living.

They are—like many of the doctors who advertise in the newspapers—trying to catch fools, so as to make a great deal of money, without thinking of the real harm they may do.

With the exception of the Dwarfs, and of some of the anecdotes, all that has been told you in this book is strictly true, and boys and girls who have read it all through, have no excuse if they do not take proper care of the wonderful little house God has given them.

If you love your parents, your country, and your God, you will try very hard to become good and healthy men and women, and to do your duty as such, at all times, and wherever you may be.

Show also that children can be trusted—as well as grown people—by never saying one word about "Nature's secret," or about any of the private parts of this book, to any one except your teacher during a lesson on this subject, or your father or mother when you are alone with them.

If your younger brothers and sisters ask you questions about these things, do not try to answer them yourself, bid them ask mother. If any of your friends wish, or need to know all that you have learned here, ask their mother's permission to lend them this book. Do not attempt to explain any part of it to any one else, for, you know, *you might* get the meaning as twisted as the rhyme I quoted to you a little while ago.

As the greatest blessings one can enjoy are a "sound mind in a sound body," do all you can to cultivate your body, mind and

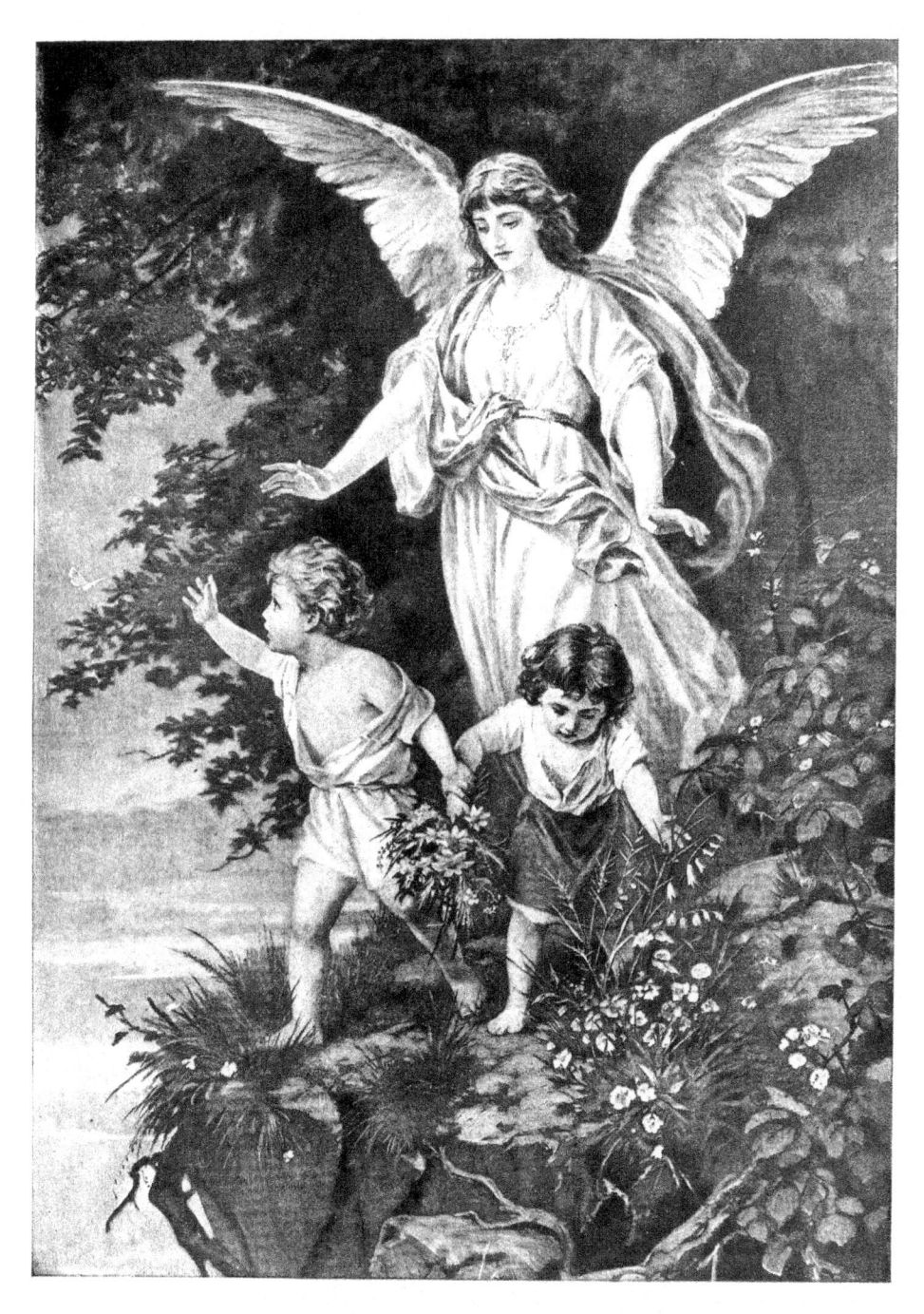

The Guardian Angel

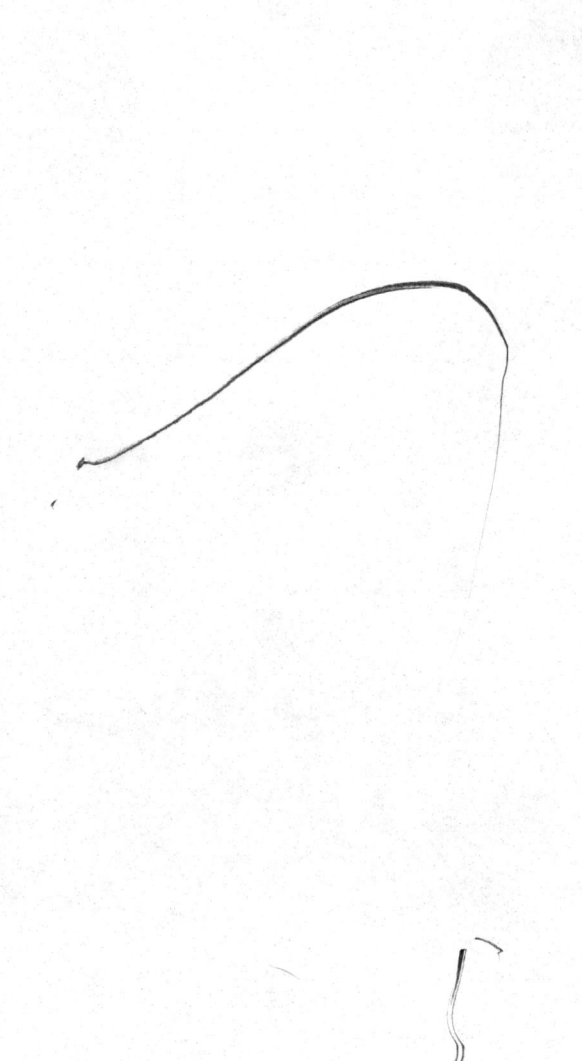

How to Get More Information 301

soul, and then you will be what God wishes you to be, and when you appear before Him, He will be able to say to you: "Well done, thou good and faithful servant."

QUESTIONS.—Do good men encourage boys to be pure? If you tried to talk about Nature's secret to anybody except your father, mother or teacher, would you be likely to make mistakes? Why should not girls read too many love stories? Is it wise to spend all your time dreaming and wishing? Why is it silly for boys and girls to pretend to be lovers? Where do girls marry very young, and what is the result? Are there pure nude pictures, and what should you do if a picture is not nice? How are you going to prove you can be trusted with "Nature's Secret," even if you are still far from grown up?

Additional titles available from
St. Augustine Academy Press

Titles by Mother Mary Loyola:

Blessed are they that Mourn
Confession and Communion
Coram Sanctissimo (Before the Most Holy)
First Communion
First Confession
Forgive us our Trespasses
Hail! Full of Grace
Heavenwards
Holy Mass/How to Help the Sick and Dying
Home for Good
Jesus of Nazareth: The Story of His Life Written for Children
The Child of God: What comes of our Baptism
The Children's Charter
The Little Children's Prayer Book
The Soldier of Christ: Talks before Confirmation
Welcome! Holy Communion Before and After

Titles by Father Lasance:

The Catholic Girl's Guide
The Young Man's Guide

Tales of the Saints:

A Child's Book of Saints by William Canton
A Child's Book of Warriors by William Canton
Illustrated Life of the Blessed Virgin by Rev. B. Rohner, O.S.B.
Legends & Stories of Italy by Amy Steedman
Mary, Help of Christians by Rev. Bonaventure Hammer
The Book of Saints and Heroes by Lenora Lang
Saint Patrick: Apostle of Ireland
The Story of St. Elizabeth of Hungary by William Canton

Check our Website for more:
www.staugustineacademypress.com

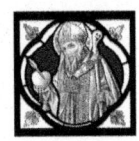

Lightning Source UK Ltd.
Milton Keynes UK
UKOW05f2043300617
304458UK00001B/97/P